AF808903

The Holistic Diverticulitis Management Guide & Cookbook

A 4-Phase Diet & Lifestyle Guide To Manage Flare-Ups, Enhance Gut Health & Well-Being

Prem Nand
Clinical Dietitian – Nutritionist

Copyright, Dedication & Legal Disclaimer

Copyright © Prem Nand, 2025

All rights reserved. No part of this book may be reproduced or used in any manner without written permission of the copyright owner except for the use of quotations in a book review. This includes photocopying of portions of the book if borrowed from a library.

First paperback edition February 2025

Book Format and Cover designed by Cindy Hyde.

Food photography by Jackie Boucher and Ariella Hoko.

For more information, please contact Prem Nand, Maximised Nutrition Ltd (publisher@maximisednutrition.com).

Published Maximised Nutrition Ltd (https://maximisednutrition.com/)

ISBN (standard paperback): 978-1-0670309-6-4
ISBN (premium paperback): 978-1-0670309-7-1
ISBN (kindle e-book): 978-1-0670309-1-9

Dedicated To:

My parents in Fiji: Vinod Kumari Nand and Nitya Nand
&
in the loving memory of my Kiwi parents: Michael & Beverley Deverell

Legal Disclaimer

This dietary and lifestyle guidance with recipes provided in this book are for educational purposes and to support you in your health journey. If you have specific dietary needs or health issues, please consult your physician or a registered dietitian for an individualized plan. For full disclaimer, go to the back page of the book.

PREFACE

Why Is Diverticular Disease An Issue?

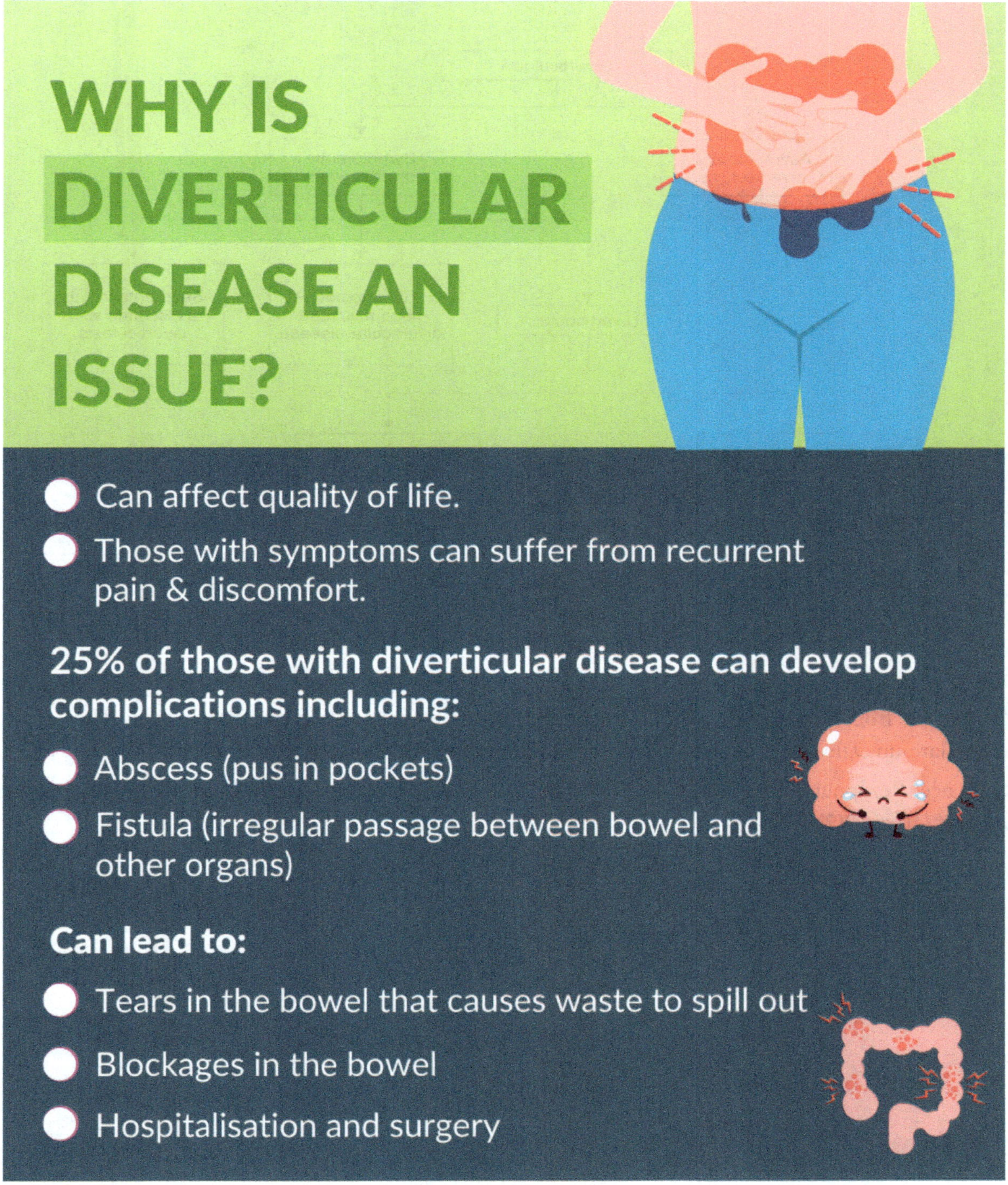

©Maximised Nutrition Ltd

Why Is A Holistic & Comprehensive Diverticular Disease Management Pathway Needed?

Answer: This has to do with the current classification of diverticular disease.

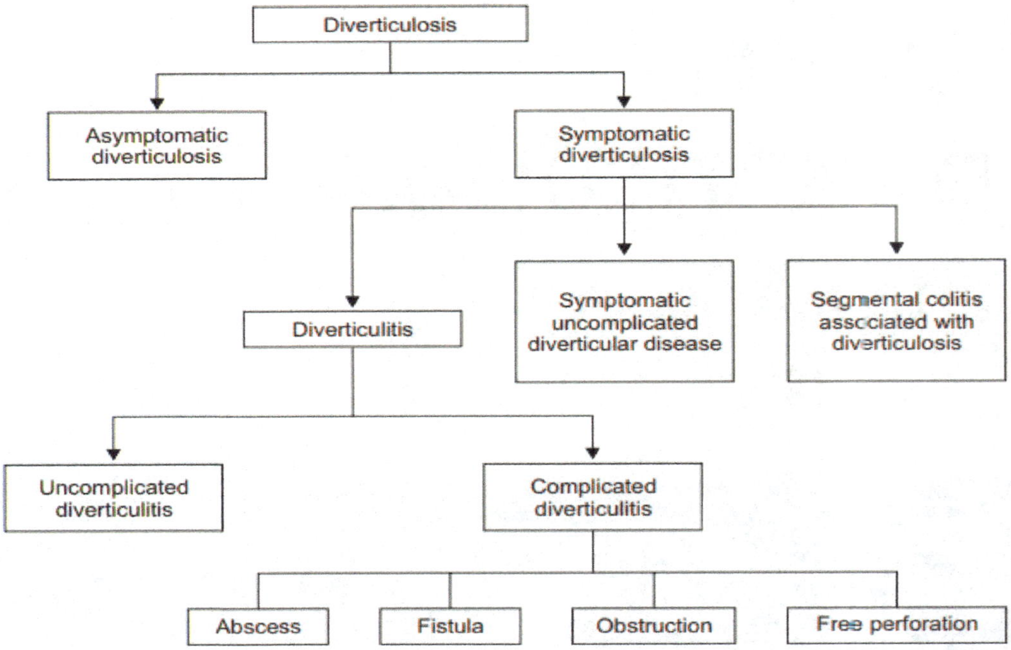

Image from Update on Pathogenesis and Management 2018

You can see from this classification flow chart the various branches of diverticular disease. Thus, the actual flare-up called diverticulitis is just one manifestation of the diverticular disease.

Reference: Rezapour, M., et al. (2018). Diverticular disease: An update on pathogenesis and management. *Gut and Liver*, 12(2), 125-132

Check If You Have Any of These Symptoms of Diverticular Disease

Some bowel symptoms can also be caused by conditions such as inflammatory bowel disease, coeliac disease, irritable bowel syndrome, or even bowel cancer. If symptoms continue, it's important to seek timely medical advice. Always consult your GP or specialist if you experience bleeding.

1. **Diverticulosis (usually symptom-free, but some people may notice the following):**
   - Mild cramps or a bit of discomfort in your abdomen
   - Feeling bloated or having a lot of gas
   - Changes in how often you go to the bathroom, either constipation or diarrhoea
   - Sometimes passing mucus when you go to the toilet
   - Mild pain, typically on the lower left side of your belly
   - Feeling like you have not fully emptied your bowels

2. **Diverticulitis (when the diverticula get inflamed or infected):**
   - Sharp, intense pain, often in the lower left part of your abdomen
   - Fever, sometimes with chills
   - Nausea or throwing up
   - Constipation, but sometimes diarrhoea instead
   - Your belly may feel tender or swollen
   - In some cases, there might be blood in your stool or bleeding from the rectum

3. **Symptomatic Uncomplicated Diverticular Disease (SUDD) (ongoing chronic unwellness)**
   - Ongoing pain, often on the lower left side of your abdomen
   - Bloating or feeling full and distended
   - Alternating between being constipated and having diarrhoea
   - Mucus in your stool
   - Feeling like you did not finish going to the bathroom
   - General discomfort, especially after eating

The symptoms of SUDD can be misdiagnosed as those of Irritable Bowel Syndrome.

4. **Diverticular Disease with SIBO/IMO (Small Intestinal Bacterial Overgrowth or Intestinal Methanogen Overgrowth):**
   - A lot of bloating and gas, especially after meals and especially after having a carbohydrate food.
   - Chronic diarrhoea, or sometimes switching between diarrhoea and constipation
   - Excessive burping or passing gas
   - Feeling tired or having difficulty concentrating (often referred to as "brain fog")
   - Symptoms related to poor nutrient absorption, like losing weight or having deficiencies
   - Abdominal pain or discomfort that tends to get worse after you eat

Symptom Checklist

SYMPTOM	Tick to indicate symptom is present	Any other comments
Discomfort in abdomen - Mild - Sharp, intense pain - On-going pain		
Feeling Bloated, with gas		
Changes to how often you go to toilet - Constipation or - Diarrhoea or - Both		
Feeling nausea or throwing up		
Passing of mucus when going to toilet		
Feeling that you have not emptied your bowels fully		
Fever, sometimes with chills		
Belly is tender or swollen		
Blood in stool		
Discomfort after eating		
Definite bloating after eating carbohydrate containing food, like bread or pasta or potato or rice		
Excessive burping of passing of wind		
Feeling tired or difficulty concentrating ("foggy brain")		
Losing weight		
Nutrient deficiencies e.g. iron deficiency		
Passing of excessive wind - Flatulence stink		

Symptom Monitoring Tool

Date	Symptoms	Details regarding what you did and what happened

Learn about Diverticulitis

Diverticulitis is an inflammation process that involves the Diverticular (pockets that form in the colon). The number of diverticular increases with age. Acute Diverticulitis can be complicated or uncomplicated.

This book will:

- help you understand the different categories of diverticular disease & their symptoms.
- teach you how to manage diverticulitis flare-ups and symptoms through diet and lifestyle through a four (4) stage management plan.
- guide you to manage each type of diverticular disease with the right diet & lifestyle plan for each stage, even when to seek help from your health care professional.
- help you adapt your everyday meals for a diverticulitis episode.
- discuss what to eat and what supplements to use to meet your recommended daily intake/allowance for nutrients.
- give you access to a 21-day menu with delicious recipes to manage stage three of your management plan.
- These menus are professionally designed and nutritionally analyzed with recommendations for portion control for meals and snacks to meet recommended daily nutrient requirements by age and gender categories for those living in Australia, New Zealand & the United States of America.
- guide you about diet & lifestyle management post-acute diverticulitis.
- Share how a particular category of diverticular can be misdiagnosed as Irritable Bowel Syndrome (IBS) and how to nutritionally manage it.
- discuss a holistic healthy eating & lifestyle guide to have during the well stage of this disease.

Holistic & Comprehensive Diet & Lifestyle Solution To Diverticular Disease

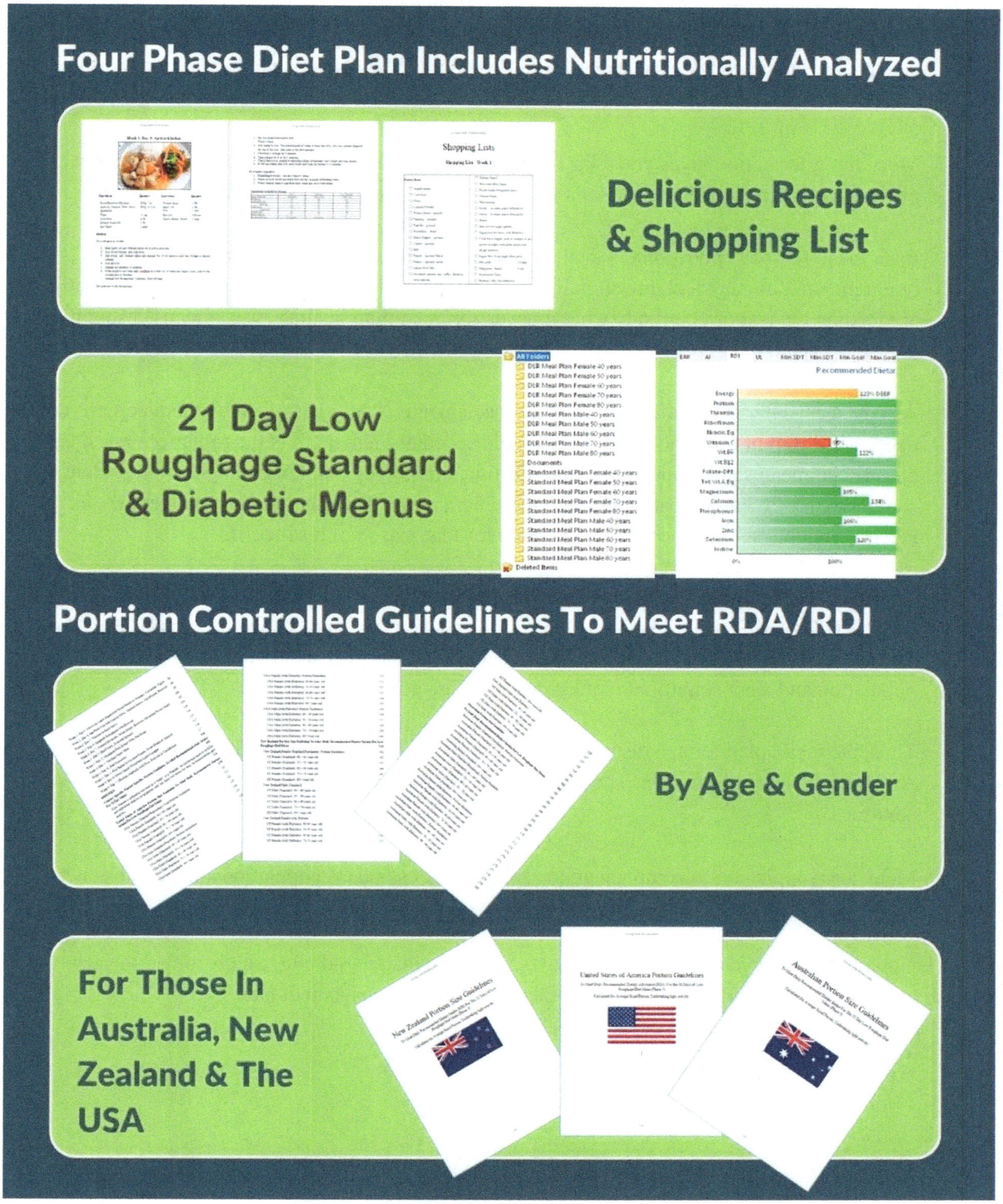

©Maximised Nutrition Ltd

What's Unique About This Nutrition Education Book?

- Most diverticulitis management plan provide a 3-stage management option. My clinical experience with patients shows that a four-stage management plan is a better option, so that patients can fluctuate between stages as needed. With the 4-stage plan, there is an opportunity to address the issues causing diverticulitis / diverticular disease to prevent recurrence, hopefully.

- Most diet information gives you a list of allowed foods and not allowed foods but does not provide a nutritionally analyzed plan that meets your Recommended Daily Requirements.

- Each menu has been nutritionally analyzed and adapted to meet a person's daily nutrient requirement. You may feel unwell in one part of your body, but you need to make sure that you are feeding the rest of your body what it needs for maximum health. These menus ensure that you are.

- As one ages, daily nutritional requirements also change. A 40-year-old active female's nutritional needs are different from those of a 70-year-old sedentary female. It is the same for males. Each decade can mean significant changes in nutritional requirements. For example, with protein, someone over 70 has a greater protein requirement per body weight than a younger person. Hence, what he /she eats needs to be adapted for that season of his /her life.

- The menu and recipes have been analyzed using country-specific nutritional values for the three countries: United States of America, Australia, and New Zealand. The nutrient profile has been compared to the recommended daily allowance / intake for that specific country and its population and against nutrient requirements for age/gender categories.

  Thus, the menu plan for an Australian 55-year-old female will be different from that of an American 55-year-old female. The information and meal plans can still be used by other countries.

- Menu and supplement recommendations are given for standard population and for those with Diabetes.

Other Unique Features have not been listed above. There are many gold nuggets given within each chapter of the book to provide the most comprehensive dietary management plan.

The Importance of Meeting Recommended Dietary Allowances / Intakes (RDAs/RDIs) Through The Menu

The 21-Day Menu (standard and diabetic versions) is designed to help meet daily nutrient needs based on Recommended Dietary Allowances (RDAs (USA)) or Recommended Dietary Intakes (RDIs (Aus/NZ)).

RDAs/RDIs aim to meet the daily nutritional requirements of 97–98% of the healthy population (FDA; Ministry of Health, AUS/NZ).

These guidelines are based on population data, where the Estimated Average Requirement (EAR) represents the median—meaning 50% of individuals need more or less (see graph below).

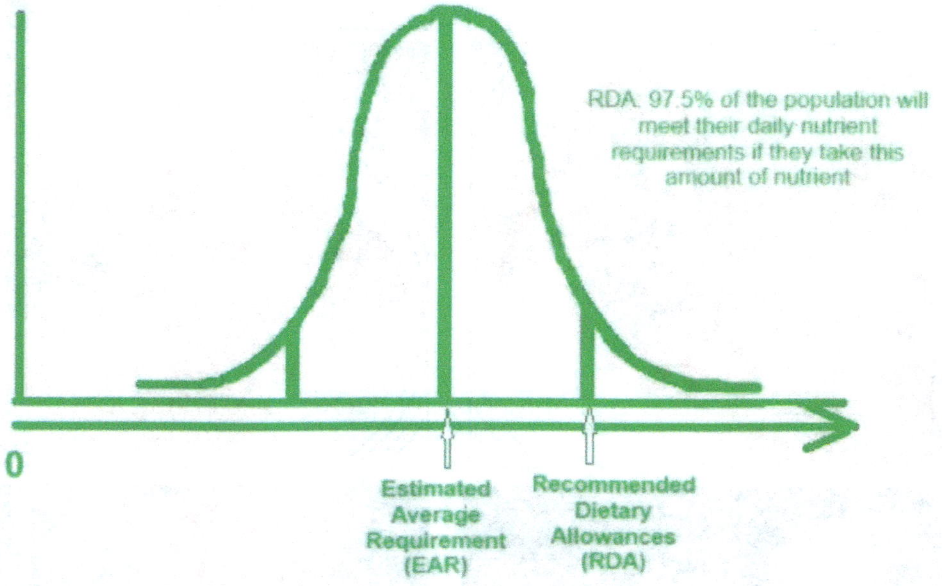

Graph: What RDAs/RDIs mean for the population

However, nutrient absorption can be impaired by gut issues, making it harder to meet individual needs through food alone.

This is particularly relevant during Phase 2 of the diverticulitis plan, which limits high-fibre foods like whole grains and legumes—potentially affecting intake of nutrients such as zinc, magnesium, selenium, and B vitamins.

It's important to monitor energy, bowel function, and overall wellbeing during each phase. Consult a registered dietitian, nutritionist, or naturopath for tailored advice if needed.

Some of the Delicious Low Roughage Recipes – Yum!

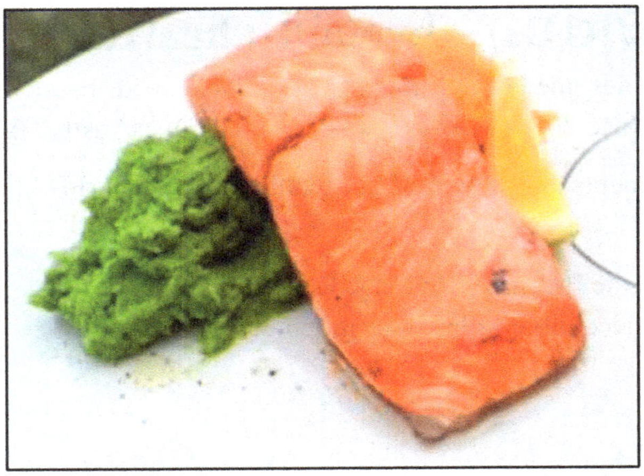

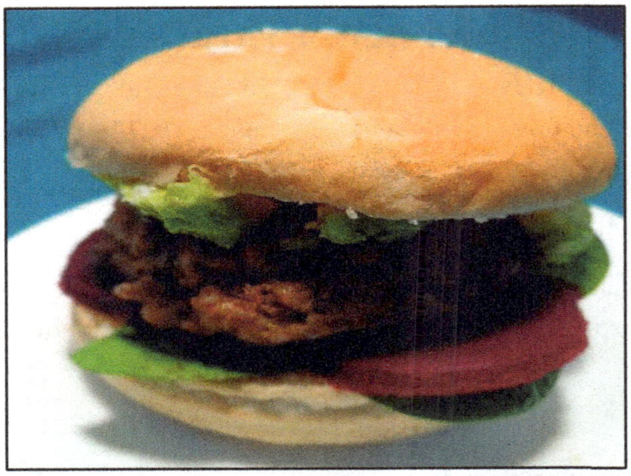

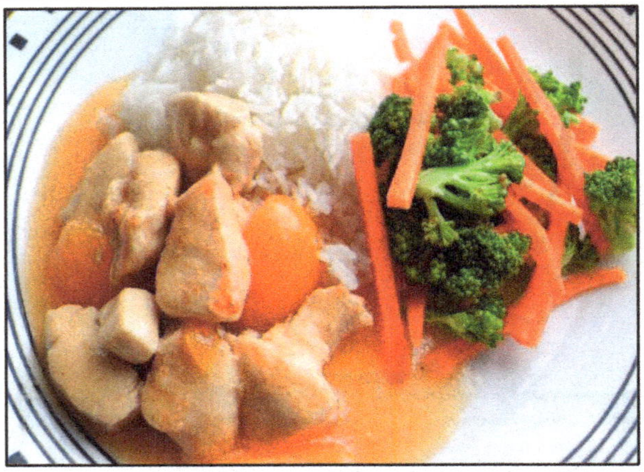

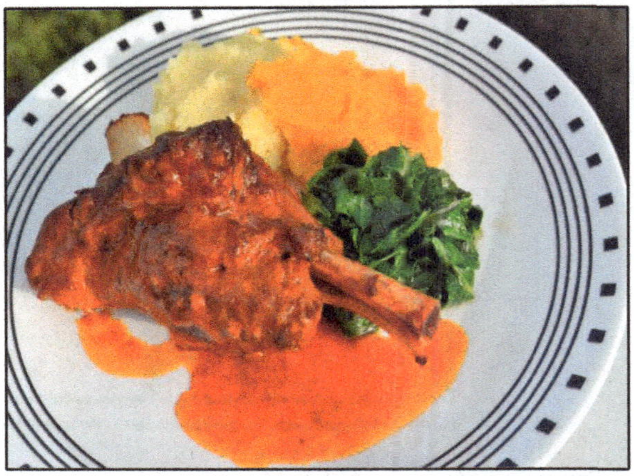

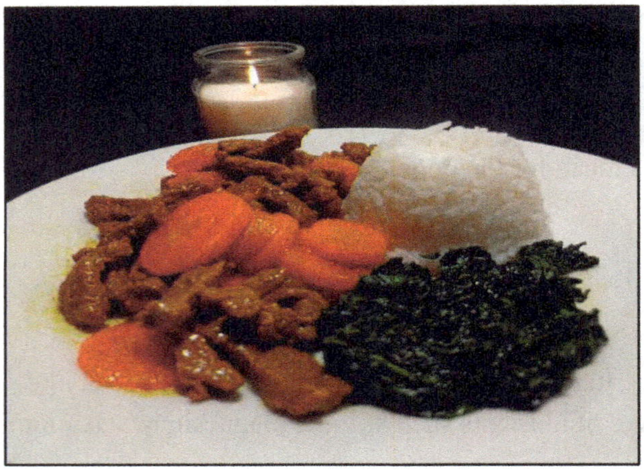

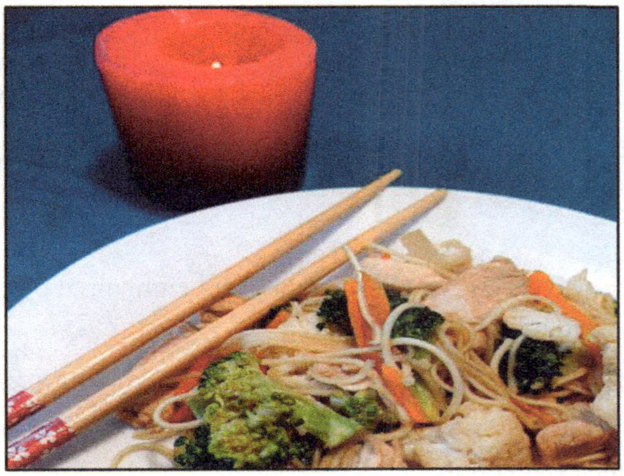

Case Studies: Diverticular Disease in Practice

The following case studies show how individualized nutrition can improve outcomes for clients with diverticular disease. Each case demonstrates different presentations and the importance of tailored intervention.

Case Study 1

A European male in his early 60s presented with fatigue, depression, insomnia, abdominal pain, and bloody diarrhea (3–4 times daily). Despite a previous hemorrhoidectomy, his GP dismissed the bleeding as hemorrhoid-related. Fear of pain and bleeding had made him avoid food.

With a history of diverticular disease, Prem Nand suspected a flare-up. Although antibiotics were recommended, the locum GP declined review. Prem started Phase 2 of the four-step guide to rest the bowel while maintaining nutrition. Within four days, bleeding stopped and bowel frequency reduced to twice daily. After one month, his energy, stool form, abdominal pain, sleep, and mental health all improved. A targeted probiotic was also added.

Case Study 2

A post-menopausal woman in her mid-60s with obesity (Level 2), depression, fatigue, and non-insulin-dependent diabetes sought support for weight loss and energy. She also reported intermittent diarrhea and abdominal pain, with a past colonoscopy confirming mild diverticular disease.

Prem designed a two-part plan: a low-roughage diabetic diet during flare-ups, and a low-GI plan with supplements to support bowel healing and microbiota balance in recovery. At six weeks, she reported higher energy, stable mood, and regular soft-formed stools. Though weight loss was minimal, she described new mental clarity. Prem advised pacing her activities to maintain progress.

Case Study 3

An elderly man in his early 80s presented with bowel incontinence, body pain, fatigue, and depression. Diagnosed with diverticular disease in his 60s, he had only been advised to take laxatives and a high-fiber diet.

Prem suspected his widespread pain was linked to nerve demyelination, confirmed by elevated homocysteine levels. He was placed on a dairy-free diet, Phase 2 of the nutrition plan, probiotics, and supplements for nerve healing. Within weeks, his stools became soft and formed, and after three months he reported reduced pain, better mood, and greater ability to manage daily tasks.

Conclusion

These cases show how diverticular disease can present in different ways. Through individualized nutritional management—bowel rest, low-GI planning, targeted probiotics, and nerve-supportive supplements—clients experienced reduced symptoms, improved bowel function, and better overall wellbeing.

About the Author

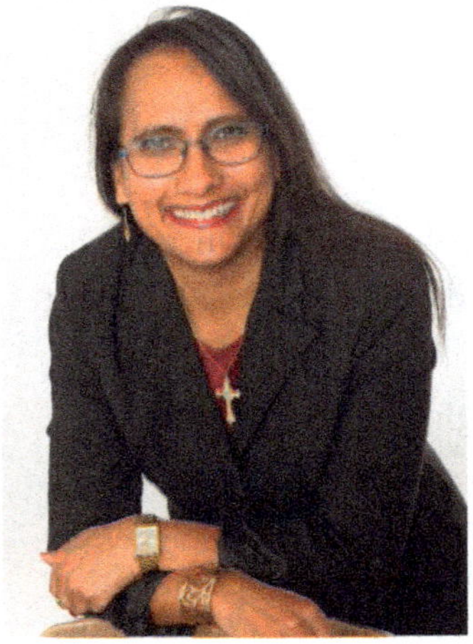

Prem Nand is a Clinical Dietitian and Nutritionist with over 20 years of experience in clinical nutrition and food service menu development. She offers consultancy services to private clients and institutions, having previously worked as a Food Service Dietitian for a regional health board. In this role, Prem developed recipes and menus for over 30 diet codes, ensuring that patients met their nutritional requirements for various medical conditions.

Her personal health journey, including recovery from a car accident and fertility challenges, fuels her passion for understanding human health and wellness. This experience drives her commitment to empowering others in their own health journeys.

Prem also holds a Diploma in Theology and resides in Whangarei, New Zealand.

Prem loves public speaking and is also involved as a leader at Girls Brigade, New Zealand.

Outside of her professional life, she enjoys her extended whanau (family & friends), fishing, gardening, and creating adventures with her daughter, embracing life as it unfolds.

Verified Google Reviews About Prem Nand's Clinical Expertise

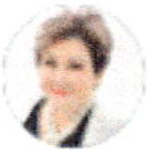

Chevaun Nel

★★★★★

I would highly recommend Prem, she has been instrumental in helping me get my health back on track!! I have a complicated medical history and there is no one size fits all with Prem she manages to tailor a plan best suited and individual to you. She has so much knowledge and experience and her advice and support has been invaluable to me. If you are looking to make positive changes in your life or have complicated medical issues you need help with, you have found the perfect person to get you started on a plan that will work for you….. and she is so lovely to work with. Thank you for everything Prem.

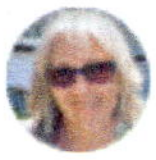

Carlysle Vivian-Robins

★★★★★

I've been working with Prem at Maximised Nutrition for a few months and would thoroughly recommend her to anybody with gut-health issues. In my initial consultation I think we both burst in to tears – mine were of total relief and joy that I was at last being heard and taken seriously after several months of symptoms including constant diarrohea, bloating, fatigue and nausea at the mere thought of food. Prem was the first person to take me seriously and shed some light on what was happening in my body and to help me work out a way forward to regaining my health. She explained everything in easy to understand terms and supported me every step of the way, making sure any changes were easily manageable within my limited budget. Her knowledge and skill are equalled by her continual thirst for new research in this area and her genuine passion for seeing people improve their quality of life.

"Hopefully, these reviews show the level of clinical expertise I bring to my practice and what I am putting into this holistic diet and lifestyle management of diverticular disease."

Prem Nand

Clinical Dietitian – Nutritionist, NZRD

Table of Contents

Chapter 1
Understanding and Managing Diverticulitis

Welcome to this holistic and comprehensive guide on understanding and managing diverticulitis. Diverticulitis is a condition where pouches called diverticula form in the wall of the intestine, often leading to discomfort and other symptoms. This chapter provides detailed information about diverticulitis, its causes, classifications, and various management strategies. Whether newly diagnosed or looking to manage your condition better, this guide will offer valuable insights into effective dietary and medical interventions.

What is Diverticulitis?

A diverticulum is a pouch that forms when the inner layer of the intestine pushes outward through a weakened part of the digestive tract's wall. This usually happens in the lower part of the large intestine. In a small part of the population, diverticula can develop in the esophagus (gullet).

Here are some terms used regarding this medical condition (Schulz et al., 2020):

Diverticula: The pouch that forms in the colon.

Diverticulosis: The presence of diverticula.

Diverticulitis: When the diverticula become inflamed (about 10 to 25% of those with diverticulosis will experience an inflammation episode in their lifetime).

Diverticular Disease: Any condition involving diverticula, whether symptomatic or asymptomatic.

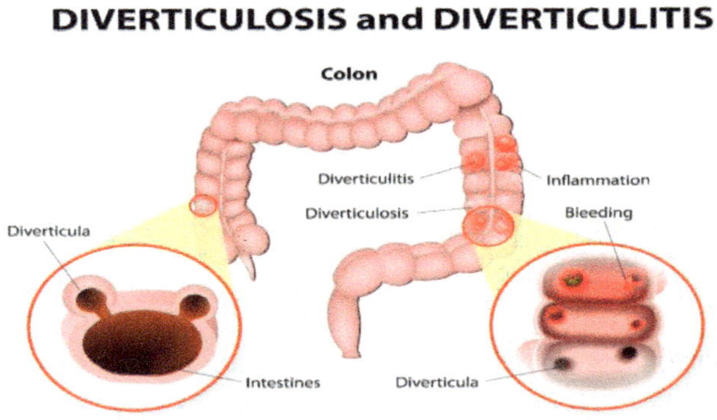

Image purchased from iStock

Classification of Diverticula Disease

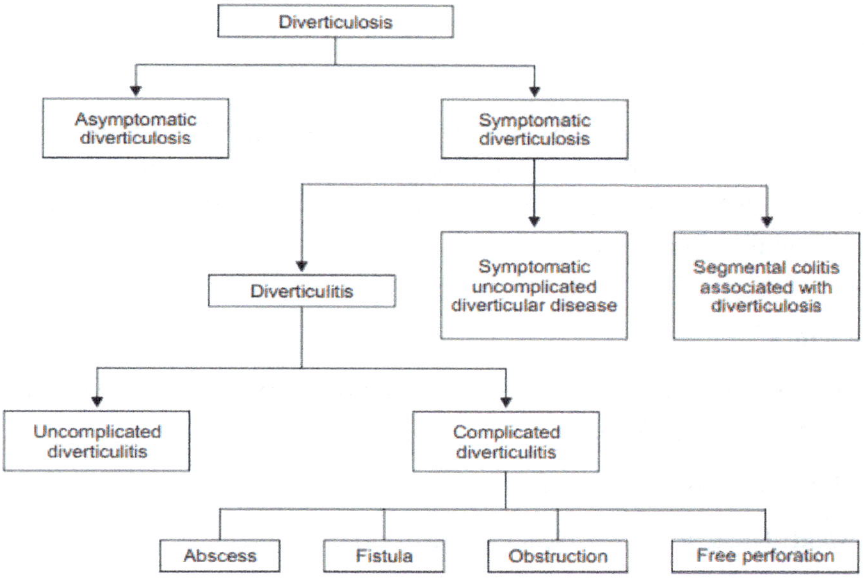

Image from Update on Pathogenesis and Management 2018 (2)

Diverticula starts forming at age 40 in both men and women. Around 10% of the population will have diverticula by the age of 40, but this increases to 50% to 70% in those over 80.

From the diagram above, if someone has diverticulosis, that they may not have any symptoms. However, around 10% to 25% of those with diverticulosis will develop diverticulitis (inflamed diverticula).

Causes of Diverticular Disease

Several factors are thought to contribute to diverticular disease.

Microbiota Involvement

The gut microbiome includes bacteria, viruses, yeast, and archaea. Normally balanced, these organisms can shift into dysbiosis, where pro-inflammatory microbes dominate. Their by-products may inflame the intestinal lining, trigger immune responses, and alter nerve function in the bowel wall. This imbalance is linked to diverticula formation (Rezapour et al., 2018).

Research shows the bacterial composition around diverticula differs from unaffected colon surfaces (Schieffer et al., 2017). This raises two possibilities: gut surface changes may promote diverticula, or existing diverticula may alter bacterial growth (Schieffer et al., 2017).

As Prem Nand (2024) notes: "Those who develop diverticulitis often have poor microbiome balance—harmful microbes lodge in intestinal pockets while impaired motility prevents waste clearance.

Inflammation weakens the gut barrier, pressure builds, and diverticular pockets form." Chapter 6 of this book further explores the role of leaky gut in diverticulitis.

Low-Fiber Diet

Traditionally, a low-fiber diet was considered a cause, as it disrupts the microbiota, reducing anti-inflammatory bacteria. However, newer studies suggest high-fiber diets may also increase diverticulitis risk (Peery et al., 2012; Yamada et al., 2015; Braunschmid et al., 2015). This highlights that diet interacts with other factors in diverticula development.

Other Risk Factors

- **High BMI:** Higher body mass, waist-to-hip ratio, or waist circumference increase risk (Braunschmid et al., 2015).
- **Smoking:** Smokers show greater incidence (Schluz et al., 2020).
- **Red Meat:** Diets rich in red meat elevate risk (Peery et al., 2012).
- **Medications:** Aspirin, NSAIDs, corticosteroids, and opiates contribute (NICE, 2019).
- **Aging Nerves:** Intestinal nerve degeneration with age may reduce bowel motility, leading to constipation, increased pressure, and diverticula (Böttner et al., 2013).

Diagnosis of Diverticular Disease

Diagnosis starts with medical history and examination (NICE, 2019). Tests include:

- **Flexible sigmoidoscopy:** Short camera tube inspects the lower intestine; biopsies may be taken.
- **Barium enema:** Barium contrast highlights the colon on X-ray to detect strictures or blockages.
- **Colonoscopy:** A long camera examines the full colon for growths, inflammation, ulcers, or bleeding; treatment may be performed during the test.
- **Virtual colonoscopy:** CT scan with contrast generates 3D colon images.
- **CT scan:** Especially useful for diverticulitis, detecting abscesses, inflammation, or perforation.

These tools confirm diagnosis and guide management.

Management of Diverticulitis

Management depends on severity (NICE, 2019; Severi et al., 2018).

- **Mild cases:** Often managed as outpatients, sometimes without antibiotics. A clear fluid or low-fibre diet is advised, with close monitoring.
- **Small abscesses (<1 cm):** Usually require hospitalization, bowel rest, IV fluids, and antibiotics.
- **Large abscesses (>1 cm):** Often need imaging-guided drainage plus IV antibiotics. Surgery may follow if unresolved.

- **Perforation and peritonitis:** Medical emergencies requiring urgent surgery, IV fluids, bowel rest, and broad-spectrum antibiotics to prevent sepsis.

Severity-based intervention improves recovery: conservative care for mild cases, intensive treatment for complicated ones.

Complications of Diverticular Disease

Diverticular disease may progress to serious complications (NICE, 2019):

- **Perforation/rupture:** Can cause abscesses or peritonitis, a life-threatening abdominal infection.
- **Diverticulitis:** Inflammation or infection of diverticula causing abdominal pain, fever, and bowel changes.
- **Bowel obstruction:** Blockages leading to pain, vomiting, and possible emergency surgery.
- **Diverticular bleeding:** Blood from a pouch appears bright red or maroon in stool and may require intervention.
- **Colitis:** Colon lining inflammation, sometimes triggered by infection or coexisting bowel disease, leading to diarrhea, pain, and bleeding.

Recognizing symptoms early enables timely treatment and better outcomes.

References

Böttner, M., Barrenschee, M., Hellwig, I., Harde, J., Egberts, J. H., Becker, T., et al. (2013). The GDNF system is altered in diverticular disease – Implications for pathogenesis. *PLoS One*, 8, e66290.

Braunschmid, T., Stift, A., Mittlböck, M., Lord, A., Weiser, F. A., & Riss, S. (2015). Constipation is not associated with diverticular disease – Analysis of 976 patients. *International Journal of Surgery*, 19, 42-45.

Jeganathan, N. A., et al. (2021). The microbiome of diverticulitis. *JGH Open*, Retrieved from https://www.sciencedirect.com/science/article/abs/pii/S2468867321000778

Prem Nand, June 2024: My explanatory comment in this book.

National Institute for Health and Care Excellence (NICE). (2019). Diverticular disease: Diagnosis and management. Retrieved from https://www.nice.org.uk/guidance/ng147

Onur, M. R., et al. (2017). Diverticulitis: A comprehensive review with usual and unusual complications. *Insights into Imaging*, 8(1), 19-27.

Peery, A. F., Barrett, P. R., Park, D., Rogers, A. J., Galanko, J. A., Martin, C. F., et al. (2012). A high-fiber diet does not protect against asymptomatic diverticulosis. *Gastroenterology*, 142, 266-272.

Rezapour, M., et al. (2018). Diverticular disease: An update on pathogenesis and management. *Gut and Liver*, 12(2), 125-132.

Schieffer, K. M., et al. (2017). The microbial ecosystem distinguishes chronically diseased tissue from adjacent tissue in the sigmoid colon of chronic, recurrent diverticulitis patients. *Microbiome*, Retrieved from https://www.ncbi.nlm.nih.gov/pmc/articles/PMC5559482

Schluz, J. K., et al. (2020). European Society of Coloproctology: guidelines for the management of diverticular disease of the colon. *Colorectal Disease*, 22(Suppl 2), 5-28. https://doi.org/10.1111/codi.15140

Severi, C., et al. (2018). Recent advances in understanding and managing diverticulitis. *F1000Research*, 7(F1000 Faculty Rev), 971. https://doi.org/10.12688/f1000research.14091.1

Yamada, E., Inamori, M., Watanabe, S., Sato, T., Tagri, M., Uchida, E., et al. (2015). Constipation is not associated with colonic diverticula: A multicenter study in Japan. *Neurogastroenterology & Motility*, 27, 333-338.

Chapter 2
Four-Phases Of Diverticulitis Management

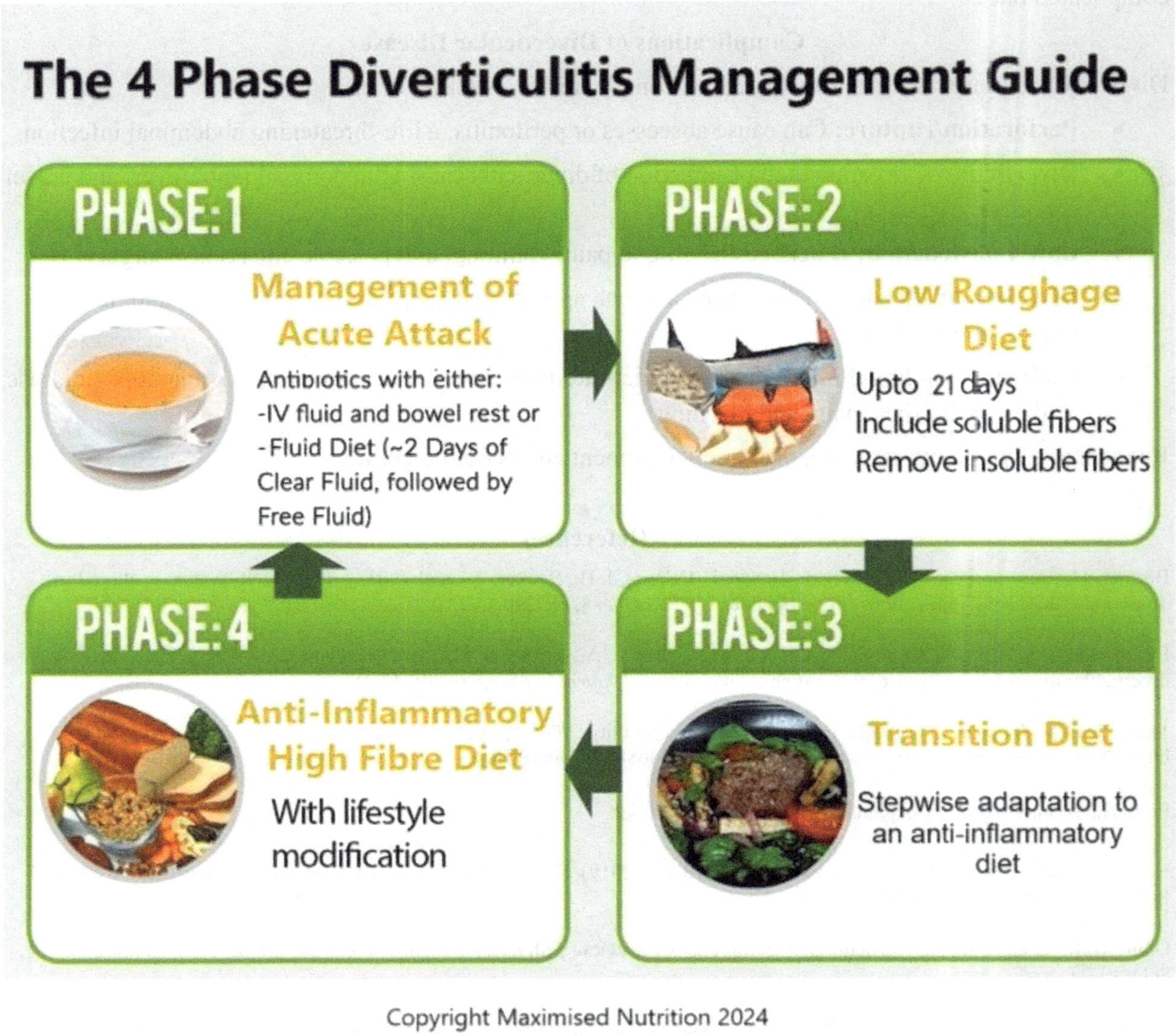

Image designed by Prem Nand, Maximised Nutrition

Phase One: Acute Management, Including The Use Of Fluid Diet

Acute management includes bowel rest with either IV fluid or a fluid diet and possibly outpatient clinic management with or without antibiotics. Severe cases may require bowel rest, IV fluids, parenteral nutrition (feeding through a tube into your vein), and surgery.

A fluid diet includes clear fluids for the initial days, followed by a free fluid diet. This can help manage symptoms and give the gastrointestinal tract a rest.

Clear Fluid Diet: Includes clear liquids that leave no residue in the intestine. Suitable for short-term use.

Free Fluid Diet: Adds milk and milk products to the clear fluid diet, providing more protein but still insufficient for long-term nutrition.

Herxheimer (Herx) Response

Note that for some patients, there will be a Herxheimer response: an acute response between a few hours to 48 hours of starting an antibiotic treatment. The reactions can have the following symptoms: headache, fatigue, tiredness, fever, chills, hyperventilation. It is thought as the bacteria is broken down, they release a substance called lipoprotein, which when absorbed into the body, can lead to an immune response (increasing inflammation). It is important to drink plenty of water / clear liquid or fluid during this time. Having extra Vitamin C may help: try clear juices like clear orange juice. Resting and getting good amounts of sleep is important too. If your blood pressure drops too low, seek medical help urgently.

Phase Two: Low Roughage Diet

This phase requires a low-roughage diet for up to 21 days, focusing primarily on soluble fiber while avoiding rough and insoluble fibers (refer to chapter 4 for in-depth information). To assist with this, the book includes a 21-day Low Roughage Menu.

Phase Three: The Transition Diet

After the 21 days of low-roughage phase, gradually introduce a high-fiber diet through a transition diet (refer to chapter 6).

Phase Four: Anti-Inflammatory High Fiber Diet

This phase of the diet is nutritionally balanced and includes adequate amounts of fiber, healthy fats, proteins, and starchy carbohydrates. I particularly enjoy following the Mediterranean Diet lifestyle, which will be explained in detail later in the book (chapters 7 & 10).

Thank you for reading this chapter. I wish you the best in your journey toward better health and well-being. Take care and stay proactive in managing your health.

Chapter 3
Phase 1: Management of Acute Attack: Introduction to Fluid Diets

Managing diverticulitis involves several steps, and understanding these phases is crucial for effective treatment. We have divided the management process into four distinct phases:

1. Management of an acute attack by resting the bowel using a fluid diet with or without use of antibiotic.
2. Low roughage diet.
3. Restricted Roughage Diet: a stepwise adaptation to a high-fiber diet.
4. Eventually, a full high-fiber diet.

This chapter will focus on the first step: the fluid diet. Understanding and implementing clear and free-fluid diets can help give your gastrointestinal tract the rest it needs during an acute diverticulitis attack. Let us dive into the specifics of these diets and how they can benefit your health.

The fluid diet consists of a clear fluid diet and a free fluid diet.

Clear Fluid Diet

A clear fluid diet includes fluids that are clear and leave no residue in the intestine after digestion. Everything in a clear, fluid diet needs to be absorbed during the digestive process. Although there is no fiber, the diet should meet the daily nutrient requirement for all nutrients except fiber.

When is a Clear Fluid Diet Used?

A clear fluid diet is used mostly when the gastrointestinal tract needs to rest for a few days. It can also be used during the management of an acute diverticulitis attack.

However, in severe cases with significant discomfort and pain, consult your doctor. It may be more appropriate to get admitted to the hospital and receive IV fluids and antibiotics.

Foods and Fluids Allowed on a Clear Fluid Diet

A clear fluid diet includes fluids that are liquid at room temperature. No solid food is allowed. Suitable options include:

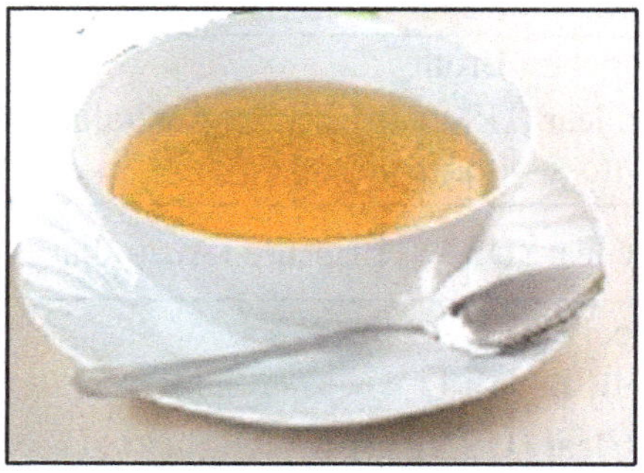

- Tea or Coffee without milk
- Clear juice including green juices (see recipe section for more details).
- Clear jelly
- Clear fizzy drinks such as lemonade
- Electrolyte sports drinks
- Clear popsicles
- Special nutritional supplements such as Ensure Clear, Diabetes Shield, or Boost Breeze (in the USA), and Ensure (in Australia and New Zealand)

Foods and Fluids Not Allowed on a Clear Fluid Diet

The following are not considered clear fluids as they leave residue or food particles behind:

- Milk
- Tomato juice
- Fruit juice with pulp
- Fruit nectar

Example of a Clear Fluid Diet

A clear fluid diet typically lasts two days. It provides only a small amount of energy and is nutrient-deficient, so it should not be used long-term.

Breakfast	Clear tea with two sugars Clear Jelly or Jell-O Ensure Clear (USA) or Ensure (Australia/ NZ)
Morning Tea	Ensure Clear (USA) or Ensure (Australia/ NZ) Ice Block Clear Green Juice
Lunch	Clear Chicken Broth Ensure Clear (USA) or Ensure (Australia/ NZ) Clear Jelly or Jell-O
Afternoon Tea	Ensure Clear (USA) or Ensure (Australia/ NZ)
Dinner	Clear Beef Broth Clear Jelly or Jell-O Ensure Clear (USA) or Ensure (Australia/ NZ)
Supper	Clear tea with two sugars

Note: This is not an endorsement of Ensure products but is used as an example of what is available in the supermarket. There may be other products around that have no residue after consumption.

The graph below (a nutritional analysis of the menu above) shows that the clear fluid diet is incomplete. Thus, it is important not to be on this diet for more than a few days.

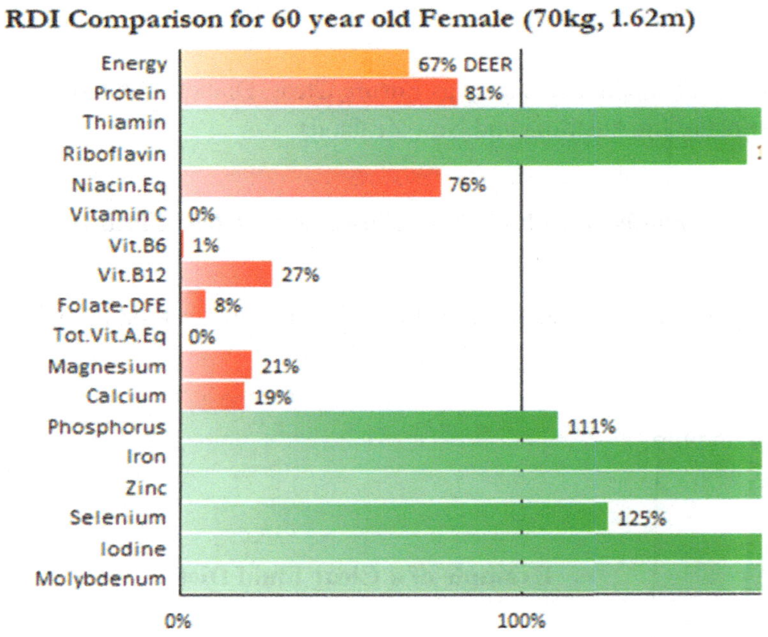

Graph: Nutritional Analysis of Clear Fluid Menu

The clear fluid menu given as an example above only provides 5003kJ Energy and 42.6g of protein.

Free Fluid Diet

After a couple of days on a clear fluid diet, you should progress to a free fluid diet. You can manage this at home but consult your GP if you experience a fever or feel unwell.

What is a Free Fluid Diet?

A free fluid diet includes all the items allowed in a clear fluid diet, plus additional items like milk and milk products. This traditionally includes:

Clear broth or Green juices	Milkshakes
Custard	Nurtitional Suppliments: Ensure Clear or Plus
Jelly or Jello	Plain ice cream
Milk	Plain yogurt

Example of a Free Fluid Diet (standard population)

Breakfast	Tea with Milk Clear Jelly or Jell-O Ensure Plus
Morning Tea	Green Vegetable Juice Plain yogurt
Lunch	Clear Chicken Broth or Clear Green Vegetable Juice Ensure Plus Clear Jelly or Jell-O
Afternoon Tea	Tea with milk Ensure Plus
Dinner	Clear Beef Broth or Clear Green Vegetable Juice Clear Jelly or Jell-O with ice cream Ensure Plus
Supper	Tea with Milk

Note: This is not an endorsement of Ensure products but is used as an example of what is available in supermarkets, e.g. Complan or Vitaplan in Australia and New Zealand.

The green vegetable juice recipes are given in section 2 under recipes.

The graph below (a nutritional analysis of the menu above) shows that the free-fluid diet is not complete. Thus, it is important not to be on this diet for more than a few days.

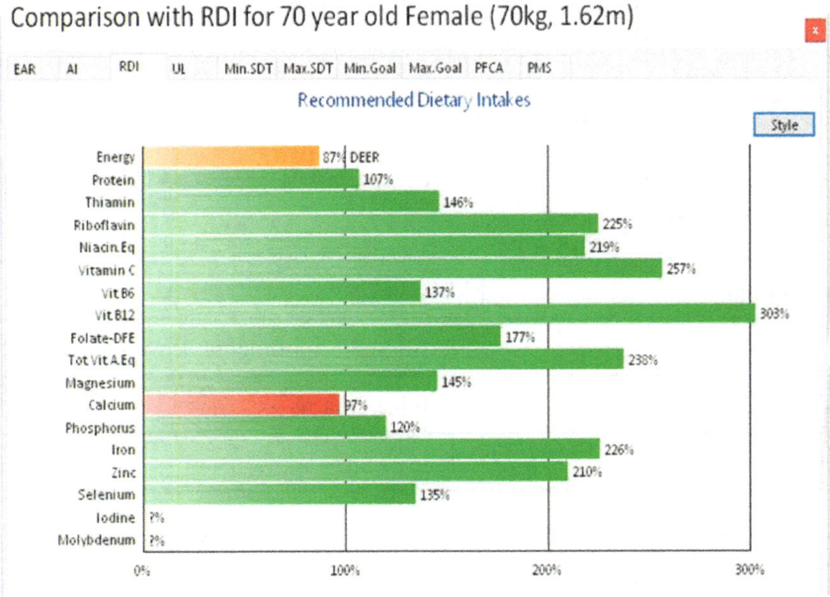

Graph: Nutritional analysis of a free fluid diet

While this diet may provide more protein if you have the right nutritional supplement, it is still insufficient in calories or nutrients for long-term use. Thus, starting on phase 3 is recommended.

Example of a Diabetic Free Fluid Diet

Breakfast	Tea with Milk Diabetic Jelly or Low Sugar Jell-O Glucerna Drink
Morning Tea	Tea with milk Plain yogurt
Lunch	Clear Chicken Broth Diabetic Jelly or Low Sugar Jell-O Glucerna Drink
Afternoon Tea	Tea with milk Glucerna Drink
Dinner	Clear Beef Broth Diabetic Jelly or Low Sugar Jell-O Low Sugar Ice Cream or Sorbet Glucerna Drink
Supper	Tea with Milk

Note: Again, this is not an endorsement of Glucerna as a product but is used as an example of what is available in supermarkets.

You can try some of the green vegetable juices given in the recipe section but check to see that your blood sugar remains within normal range 2 hours after a drink (just to make sure you do not get a hypoglycemic response. I do not think you will but I recommend the side of precaution).

The graph below (a nutritional analysis of the menu above) shows that the free-fluid diet is not complete. Thus, it is important not to be on this diet for more than a few days.

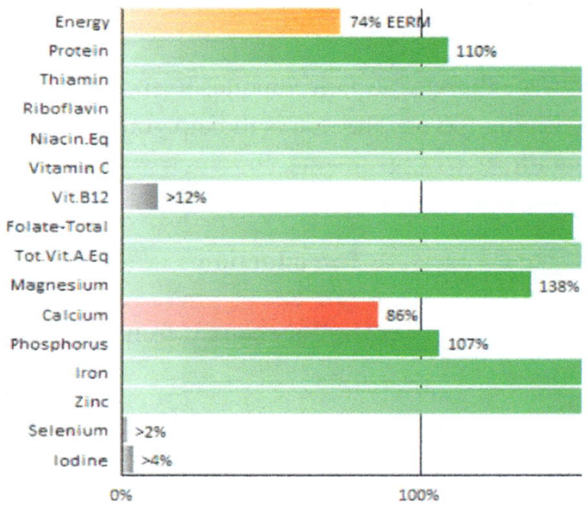

Graph: Nutritional analysis of a diabetic free fluid diet

Summary

This chapter has provided valuable insights into managing diverticulitis through the implementation of fluid diets. By understanding the clear and free-fluid diets, you can give your gastrointestinal tract the rest it needs during an acute attack, allowing for a smoother recovery process.

Remember, these dietary adjustments are essential to managing diverticulitis, but they should be tailored to your individual needs. Always consult your GP for personalized advice and guidance. Clear and free fluid diets are designed to be short-term solutions that provide relief and aid in the healing process.

As you progress through these dietary phases, remember the importance of listening to your body and adjusting as necessary. This knowledge empowers you to take control of your condition and improve your quality of life. Stay proactive, stay informed, and, most importantly, stay healthy.

Thank you for reading this chapter. I hope you find these guidelines helpful and supportive in your journey toward better health and well-being. Take care and continue to prioritize your health as you navigate the challenges of living with diverticulitis.

Chapter 4
Phase 2: Introduction To A Low Roughage Diet

In this chapter, I will show you practical ways to adapt your everyday foods, making them suitable for a low-roughage diet. This diet is beneficial for managing diverticulitis and helps with conditions like ulcerative colitis and more.

We will cover everything from meal preparation techniques to specific ingredient substitutions that reduce roughage without sacrificing flavor. The aim is to help you enjoy your meals and live life fully while making these simple yet effective adjustments.

Introduction

In acute stage, those suffering from diverticulitis may benefit from a clear fluid diet with antibiotics for up to two days.

Clear fluid diet includes jelly, clear juice, clear broths, and clear nutritional supplements such as Ensure Clear.

As the inflammation is brought under control, a free fluid diet may be initiated.

After this, a low roughage diet that is low in insoluble fiber or resistant starch is introduced. The aim of a low roughage diet is to keep the fecal bulk to a minimum so that there is not a lot of pressure on the affected area.

A low roughage diet is recommended for up to 21 days after which a transition to a high fiber diet is recommended.

What Is A Low Roughage Diet?

Dietary fiber is a group of carbohydrates that cannot be digested by the enzymes that break down carbohydrate. They are found in fruit, vegetables, nuts, lentils, legumes, and grains.

There are three forms of fiber: insoluble fiber (does not dissolve in water), soluble fiber (which dissolves in water) and resistant starch.

Sources of soluble fiber are: rolled oats, peeled apples, carrots, barley.

Sources of insoluble fiber include nuts, whole grain, unbroken grains, fibrous parts of cauliflower, cabbage, broccoli etc.

A diet can be high in soluble fiber but low in insoluble fiber (This diet is called a low roughage diet).

In case of diverticulitis, in the transition phase from fluid diet to high fiber diet, it is recommended a balanced diet low in insoluble fiber (or Low Roughage Diet) is followed for a short period of time (for up to 21 days) after an acute inflammatory episode.

Recent research does not support avoidance of nuts and seeds during well stage. One preventative habit is to chew all food in the mouth till it is smooth. Maximised Nutrition Limited is a bit more cautious and advises that if patient experience shows that symptoms of flare are related to certain foods, then avoid these foods.

Note: Many of the diverticulitis management diet plans talk about a low residue diet. This is not the approach I take.

A low roughage diet is different from a low residue diet. A low residue diet means that there is minimum residue or bulk left after fiber is digested. A low roughage diet, however, takes out the gritty, undigestible fibers from the diet (the parts that could irritate an inflamed gut surface) but allows bulk to be formed after digestion is completed.

We still want fiber so that we can feed the gut microbiome, but we want them to be high in soluble fiber (leaving minimum residue in the gut).

Adapting Common Food to A Low Roughage Option

We can use certain foods that have insoluble fiber by adapting how we prepare them for cooking and consumption. Below are some examples.

Flavoring with Low Roughage

Garlic and Onion

Garlic and Onion add deliciousness to our cooking. Normal garlic is high in roughage, but you can pound it and filter out the rough parts using a sieve. You can make your own flavored oils using onion and garlic.

Step 1: Pound or fine-chop onion or garlic.
Step 2: Add to a cup of oil in a pot.
Step 3: Simmer to extract oil.
Step 4: Allow to cool
Step 5: Use a sieve and extract flavored oil. Discard tough fibers.
Step 5: Pour into a sterilized, airtight glass bottle and use for cooking as needed.

Italian Herb Infused Oil

For this you need:

1 cup of Olive Oil
6 leaves of basil
2 sprigs (around 1 tablespoon) of fresh thyme
2 sprigs (around 1 tablespoon) of fresh rosemary
2 sprigs (around 1 tablespoon) of fresh oregano

(if you do not have fresh herbs, pound 1 tsp each of the above using mortar and pestle with some oil).

Add the above to the cup of olive oil. And place in an air-tight bottle. Use within 2 to 3 days. I like to leave this for a day to allow the herbs to infuse into the oil. When using the herb infused oil, just use the oil, sieving off the herb part of it.

This is great to use in the homemade creme of tomato soup.

Indian Spice Infused Oil

For this recipe, you will need the following:

3 tablespoons whole coriander seeds
2-3 whole cloves
2 tablespoons whole cumin seeds
1 two-inch piece cinnamon stick (break into smaller bits)
10 whole green cardamom pods
5 bay leaves or curry leaves (curry leaves are different from bay leaves).
1 tablespoon ground turmeric
2 cup olive oil

1. In a heavy bottomed pan, add the cumin seeds, the coriander seeds, cinnamon sticks, whole cloves.
2. Lightly toast for two minutes. Remove from heat.
3. Place in a grinder or a pastel and motor and grind to fine powder.
4. Add these with turmeric and bay leaves in oil and put in an air tight bottle. It can keep for two weeks.
5. Before using it for cooking, use a fine sieve and remove any debris or residue.

Vegetable Preparation

Brocolli Cut the florets to reduce fiber content. Boil to soften. 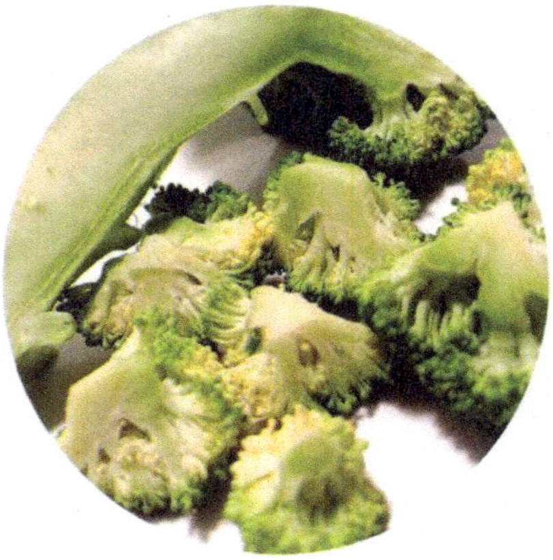	**Cauliflower** You can make a puree by boiling or steaming, then blending smooth. 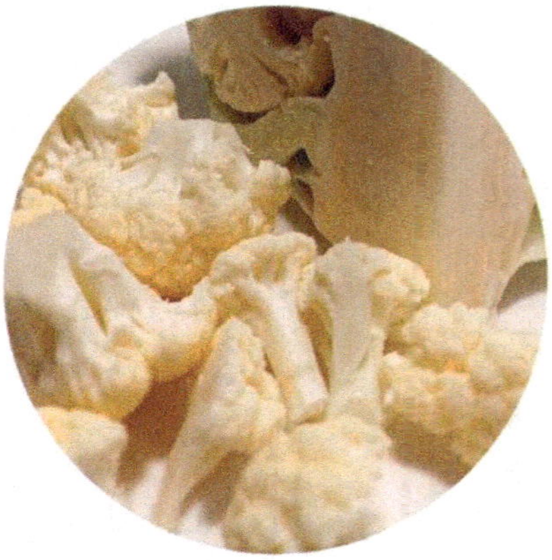

Zucchini and Cucumber Peel the skin off and remove the seeds to make them low roughage. Eat only the white flesh. 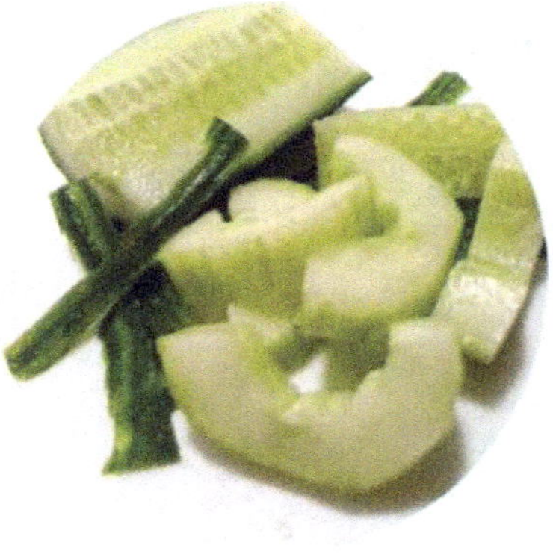	**Pumpkin** Remove the skin. Boil, steam, or microwave instead of roasting to keep the fiber soft. If roasting, cook until done but not caramelized. 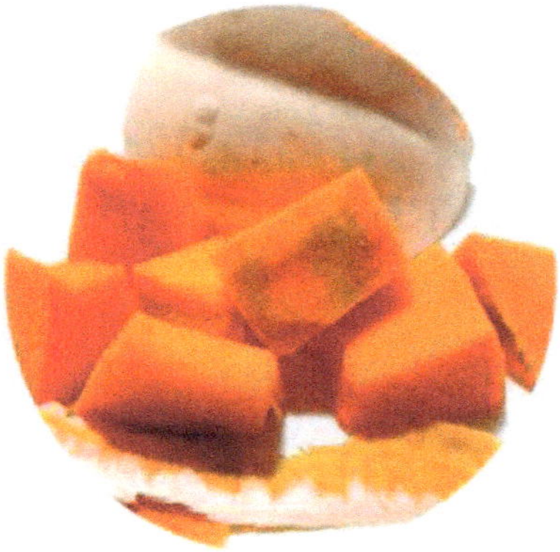

Silverbeet (Swiss Chard) 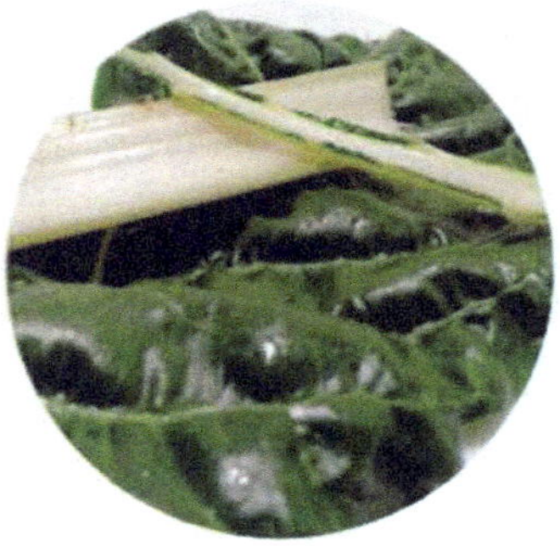	Use the leaves and cut off the white stems to reduce roughage content.

Fruit Preparation

Apple or Pear 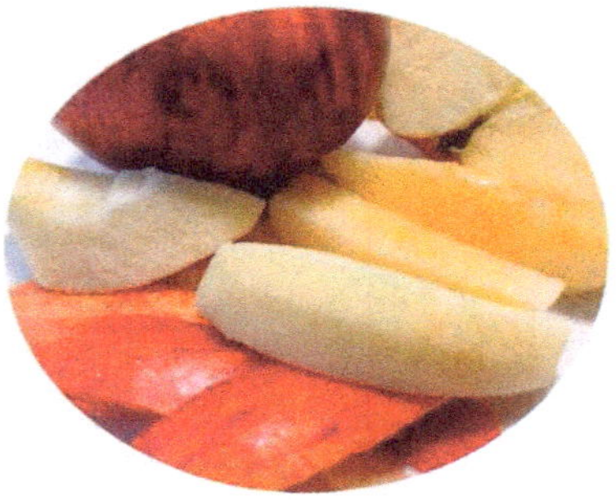	Remove the skin and seeds. Stew the apple for easier digestion and bottle it in sterilized containers for food safety.

Snack Options

Fruit Rolls or Plain Muffins

Choose soft fruit rolls without seeds. Plain fine flour muffins such as chocolate muffins, vanilla muffins, Madeira cake or sponge cakes are okay.

Herbs and Seasonings

Onion, Garlic, and Parsley

Use a pastel and mortar to pound them to extract essential oils and flavors, making them easier to digest. Then, use a sieve to remove the extract and discard the fiber.

Cumin

Ground cumin is preferable to whole seeds for a low roughage diet.

Soups

Cream Soups 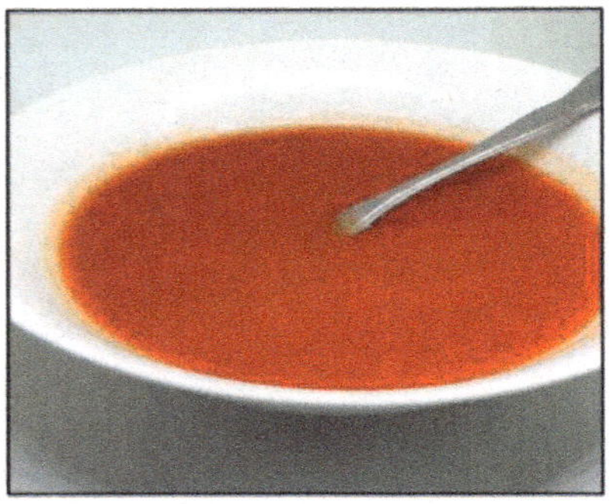	Make your soups or choose cream soups from the supermarket. Use a sieve to remove any roughness before consuming.

Table: Suitable Food Types and Foods Types to Avoid When On A Low Roughage Diet

Category	Suitable Types	Types to Avoid
Bread	White Bread or toast (Oatilicious) Fine Wholemeal Bread High fiber White Bread, English Muffins	Breads with unbroken seeds, whole grains, nuts, kibble wheat Burned or crusty toast
Cereals	Fine Rolled Oats Cornflakes or Rice Bubbles White Rice, Pasta, Sago, Tapioca Cornflour, White Flour	Bran, Muesli, All Bran, Wholemeal Flour, Wholemeal or Whole Grain Pasta, Brown Rice, Wheat Germ Caution with Doughy Foods such as Scones, Very Fresh Bread
Cakes / Biscuits	Plain Sweet Biscuits Ginger Nuts, Shortbread, Rice Cakes, Rice Wafers, Plain Sponge Cakes, Madeira Cake	Wholemeal or bran biscuits, cakes or biscuits with dried fruit, nuts, coconut
Desserts	Jello, Plain desserts, milk puddings yogurt, plain ice cream	Any containing seeds, skins, coconuts, nuts, dried fruit
Fruit	Fruit without skin or seeds such as melon, pawpaw, banana, apples, pears, peaches	Fruit with pips, skin or seeds such as Kiwifruit, strawberries, cranberry, citrus pith and membrane, dried fruit such as figs, sultanas, raisins, currents
Vegetables	Soft vegetables without tough fibers or skins e.g. - Skinless potato, Skinless kumara - Skinless and seedless pumpkin - Skinless beetroot - Soft leaves of Swiss Chard (no stems) - Peeled carrots - Cauliflower tips - Broccoli tips	Corn, baked beans, peas, seeds, skins, pips or course stalks, mushroom, cabbage family, onion, garlic, tomato, beans, broad beans Roasted Vegetables, Fried Chips
Nuts / Seeds	Smooth peanut butter Nutella Finely ground nuts	Crunchy peanut butter Nuts: whole, chopped Sesame seeds, sunflower, poppy or pumpkin seeds
Beverages	Weak tea or coffee. Infused Fruit Flavored Tea. Clear Fruit Juice or Vegetable Juice or Cordial	Fruit Drinks with Pulp
Dairy	All varieties of milk Plain yogurt or custard Plain or flavored ice-cream Cheese	Any containing died fruit, nuts or coconut Shakes etc that have chunky fruit or vegetable pieces Cheeses with nuts or seeds, fruit yogurt with seeds, skins
Fat	All plain spreads or fat such as butter, margarine, cream, oil, plain salad dressing	Rich mayonnaise, rich pastry, batter, fried foods
Meat, Fish, Poultry, Eggs, Nuts, Legumes	Tender meat, fish, poultry, lean bacon or ham. Meat or fish paste, smooth spreads, poached eggs	Tough grisly meats, fried or highly seasoned or herbed meat or meat products e.g. sausages, prepared dried meats such as jerky, fried eggs
Others	Plain gravy Lollies, sugar, honey, plain ice cream toppings	Pop corn

Chapter 5
Introduction to the 21-Day Low Roughage Menu

In this chapter, I will explain how I developed this menu and how you can effectively manage your diverticular disease. We will cover everything from portion sizes tailored to different countries and age groups to specific dietary needs for those with diabetes. Remember, this menu is designed to help you enjoy your meals while managing your condition, ensuring you get the proper nutrients without compromising taste or enjoyment. Let us dive in and explore how these simple adaptations can make a big difference in your daily diet.

For recipes to support all your phases, please refer to section three.

What is the 21-Day Low Roughage Menu?

This section outlines the 21-day low roughage menu for people with diverticular disease. The menu is created for a standard, healthy population and has also adapted for those with diabetes.

Suitability of the Menu

If you have multiple health problems, this menu may not be suitable. In this case, please consult with your health professional. However, it is primarily designed for individuals with diverticular disease. The menu provides information on portion sizes guideline for those living in the United States of America, Australia, and New Zealand by gender and age categories.

Age Categories and Nutritional Requirements

The menu is divided into the following age categories:

- 40 to 50
- 50 to 60
- 60 to 70
- 70 to 80
- 80+

These categories exist because nutritional requirements vary with age. For example, a person over 65 will have higher protein needs than someone in a lower age category.

Country-Specific Considerations

Different countries have different food sources, such as variations in bread ingredients and meat cuts. These differences affect the protein amounts in the meat. The average heights and weights of the population for different countries also differ by age categories. For example, an average 40-year-old to 49-year-old USA female weighs 67kg and has a height 1.62m. An average 40 year to 49-year-old

Australian female weighs 71kg and has a height 1.62m. On the other hand, an average New Zealand female weighs 68kg and has a height 1.65m.

Therefore, the menu is analyzed to meet the daily nutritional requirements for the three countries (Australia, New Zealand, and USA) by age and gender (male and female) category. Note though, the nutrition education information and recipes and menus can be used by other countries. The Author only had the analysis program for the three above named countries.

Nutrient Analysis

The data revealed that following the menu using the specified portion sizes will meet the nutritional requirements for most nutrients. However, some subgroups may still lack certain nutrients, which will be discussed in a later section on nutritional supplementation.

Nutritional Differences by Age and Gender

The menus are analyzed to ensure compliance with the recommended daily intake of particular nutrients. For example, following the diet for a female diabetic aged 40 to 50 may result in lower vitamin C intake compared to other age groups. Another example is where a 40-year-old to 50-year-old male needs more calories than a female of the same age, just because of their physical makeup.

Nutritional Supplementation

In a later section, we will discuss the use of multivitamins or other supplements to address potential nutrient deficiencies identified in the analysis. I hope this introduction to the 21-day low roughage menu has been enlightening and helpful. Understanding how to adapt your meals to meet your dietary needs allows you to manage your diverticular disease more effectively while still enjoying delicious and nutritious food.

Go to section 4 for country specific, age specific, gender specific daily meal portion guidelines for the 21 days.

Comments on the Diabetes Menu

Blood sugar levels can increase during flare-up. Thus, the Diabetes menu has been designed to help those with diabetes balance their protein and carbohydrate during the day to regulate the blood sugar level.

Keep a record of your blood sugar reading: half an hour before a meal and 2 hours after a meal if possible and adjust your insulin or medications as needed.

Can You Have Biscuits, Cakes, Muffins etc. As Snacks?

You can have plain biscuits, plain muffins, scones etc. but the way I designed this guide and menus is to is to ensure that a) you are meeting at least the recommended daily dietary requirements. B) that your gut microbiome has the best chance of recovering to optimal balance. Feeding refined sugar products potentially can lead to the pathogenic microbiome growing in greater numbers than the beneficial microbiome. By not feeding refined sugar products and increasing intake of prebiotics (found in fruit and vegetables, like the use of green smoothies), you can help the beneficial microbiome to establish well in the gut ecosystem. So I would caution about having biscuits, cakes, muffins etc for snacks in the phases 2 & 3 but introduce them when you doing high fiber diet, as part of normal healthy eating plan.

Chapter 6
Phase 3: Transition Phase

Now that you have done 21 days of Low Roughage Diet, I hope that your discomfort and symptoms have improved. If you wish to stick to a low roughage diet for a few more days or another week, do so. However, it is time to implement the transition phase.

This phase is up from a low roughage menu but it still avoids hard, undigestible insoluble fibers. This diet is aiming to get you to a high fibre diet eventually.

The Transition Phase Diet

This diet avoids course and hard to digest foods such as pips, seeds, nuts, skins, wholegrain breads and cereals, "stringy" foods such as celery, rhubarb, vegetables such as corn, baked beans, citrus fruits (with its segment covering), and tough meats.

New foods should be introduced one at a time and in small quantities. If a new food upsets your gut, avoid it for 3 to 4 weeks, then try again.

Some pointers:

- Eat slowly and chew foods well
- Eat regularly, as skipping meals may cause problems with flatulence and constipation.
- You can start to introduce more roughage in your diet through your smoothies: use the fruit and vegetable from the list below. No need to just have fruit juices. Having more roughage will feed those gut microbiome.
- Continue with your probiotics but can stop pre-biotic tablets/capsules as the fiber from the food will now provide more of the prebiotics. Foods rich in pre-biotics include onion, garlic, Yacon roots or cassava, banana skin, flax seed (use ground version), dandelion greens, barley, buckwheat. Onion can cause flatulence so introduce this by itself as a new food in the existing diet for a few days and monitor your symptoms.
- Remember to read the chapter on SUDD and SIBO/IMO. If your gut has too much bloating, causes reflux, etc, then this list may not be appropriate for you. I suggest consult with a Clinical Dietitian – Nutritionist or a naturopath to get further investigations and an individualized nutrition plan.

Chapter 7
Phase 4: Best Diet When Well Recovered

Now that you are well, it is crucial that we establish a great gut health. You may already know that gut microbiomes affect every part of your body.

Prem Nand's Recommendation for The Best Diet for Your Gut & Well-Being

I am of the view that the Mediterranean Diet is the best overall diet for your health (unless you are suffering from Sudden Uncomplicated Diverticular Disease (SUDD) or SIBO/IMO complication of diverticulitis (see the chapters following this one). However, Prem Nand still recommends avoiding hard insoluble fiber foods such as unbroken nuts, seeds, corn unless it is chewed to smooth paste in your mouth during this well phase.

The high-fiber Mediterranean diet is renowned for its health-promoting properties. It offers a wide range of benefits, including anti-inflammatory effects, improved gut microbiome health, and enhanced brain function. This dietary pattern is based on the traditional eating habits of countries bordering the Mediterranean Sea, emphasizing nutrient-dense, minimally processed foods.

Core Components of the Mediterranean Diet

A Mediterranean diet is rich in monounsaturated fats, primarily from olive oil and avocados, and omega-3 fatty acids from fish like salmon, mackerel, and sardines. Lean proteins such as chicken and plant-based options like legumes (lentils, chickpeas) and nuts are staples. Green vegetables like spinach, kale, and broccoli are abundant, complemented by whole grains, fruits, and herbs. Coconut oil, though less traditional, is sometimes included for its medium-chain triglycerides, which support energy metabolism.

Anti-Inflammatory Properties

The diet's anti-inflammatory effects are mainly attributed to its high omega-3 fatty acids, polyphenols, and dietary fiber content. Omega-3 fatty acids in fatty fish modulate inflammatory pathways by influencing eicosanoid production (Calder, 2010). Polyphenols from olive oil and green vegetables act as antioxidants, reducing oxidative stress and inflammation (Farràs et al., 2013). The fiber in whole grains and vegetables promotes a healthy gut microbiota, further reducing systemic inflammation (Rinninella et al., 2019).

Benefits for the Gut Microbiome

The Mediterranean diet fosters a diverse and robust gut microbiome. Dietary fiber from vegetables, fruits, and whole grains acts as a prebiotic, feeding beneficial bacteria like *Bifidobacteria* and *Lactobacilli*. These bacteria produce short-chain fatty acids (SCFAs), such as butyrate, which strengthen the gut barrier and reduce inflammation (Koh et al., 2016). A healthier gut microbiome is linked to reduced risks of metabolic disorders, obesity, and colorectal cancer (Tilg et al., 2020).

Cognitive and Brain Health

Research shows that the Mediterranean diet supports cognitive function and protects against neurodegenerative diseases. The antioxidants in polyphenol-rich foods reduce oxidative damage in the brain, while omega-3s support neuronal health and improve memory and learning (Estruch et al., 2013). Moreover, SCFAs from a fiber-rich diet have neuroprotective effects, potentially reducing risks of Alzheimer's disease and depression (Bienenstock et al., 2015).

Conclusion

A high-fiber Mediterranean diet is a cornerstone of holistic health. Its anti-inflammatory effects, gut microbiome benefits, and cognitive advantages make it a powerful approach to enhancing overall well-being.

"There are times when I will modify the Mediterranean Diet to individualize the diet for a client, depending on other presenting medical issues but I mostly use the concepts of the Mediterranean diet in my practice," Prem Nand, Clinical Dietitian – Nutritionist.

Refer to chapter 10 on more tips on healthy diet and lifestyle choices to prevent recurrence of diverticulitis flare-ups.

References

Calder, P. C. (2010). Omega-3 fatty acids and inflammatory processes. *Nutritional Research Reviews*.

Farràs, M., et al. (2013). Polyphenols and anti-inflammatory pathways. *Molecular Nutrition & Food Research*.

Rinninella, E., et al. (2019). Gut microbiota and diet: Implications in health and disease. *Nutrients*.

Koh, A., et al. (2016). Short-chain fatty acids and gut health. *Nature Reviews Gastroenterology & Hepatology*.

Tilg, H., et al. (2020). Gut microbiome in health and disease. *Nature Reviews Gastroenterology & Hepatology*.

Estruch, R., et al. (2013). Mediterranean diet and cognitive function. *New England Journal of Medicine*.

Bienenstock, J., et al. (2015). The gut-brain axis and SCFAs. *Nature Reviews Gastroenterology & Hepatology*.

Chapter 8
Understanding Symptomatic Uncomplicated Diverticular Disease (SUDD)

In this chapter, I want to discuss a subclass of diverticular disease that is often overlooked: symptomatic uncomplicated diverticular disease (SUDD). In the first few chapters, we covered a wide range of diverticular conditions, including symptomatic and asymptomatic cases and both complicated and uncomplicated diverticulitis.

Let us now focus on SUDD and its role in chronic inflammation syndrome.

SUDD is a persistent yet often misunderstood condition. Many patients experience ongoing discomfort, such as diarrhea, bloating, irregular bowel movements, gas, and pain, which are frequently misdiagnosed as irritable bowel syndrome (IBS).

However, these symptoms can persist even in the absence of visible inflammation.

Recognizing and correctly diagnosing SUDD is crucial for effective management and improving patient quality of life. This chapter will delve into the causes, current research, and practical treatment options, including dietary adjustments, to help you better understand and manage SUDD.

What is SUDD?

Symptomatic uncomplicated diverticular disease (SUDD) is characterized by persistent abdominal symptoms attributed to diverticula without obvious colitis or diverticulitis. Essentially, there is no visible inflammation, but symptoms such as diarrhea, bloating, irregular bowel movements, gas, and ongoing pain persist even after antibiotic treatment. Often, these symptoms are misdiagnosed as irritable bowel syndrome (IBS), but they indicate SUDD.

Understanding Chronic Inflammation Syndrome

To understand SUDD, it is essential to understand the structure of your bowel and how it functions.

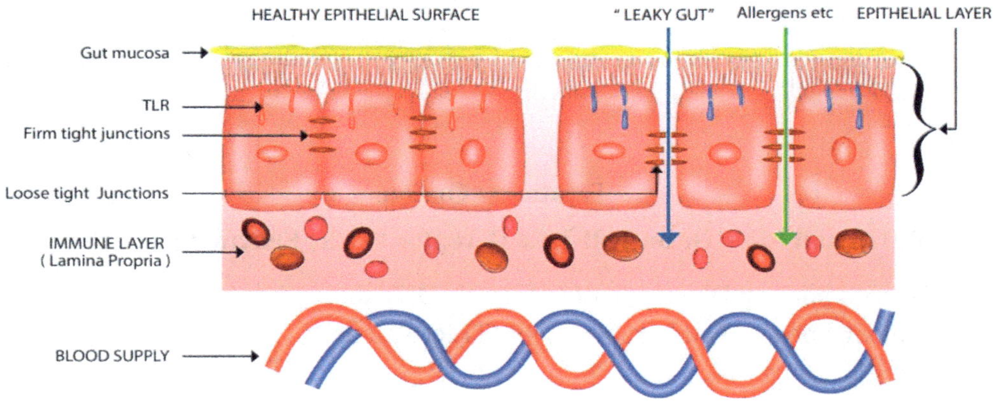

Your colon has a thin layer of epithelial cells that separate the intestinal contents from the rest of your body. This epithelial layer is protected by a mucus layer, which acts as a barrier against acids, chemicals, and food particles. There are toll-like receptors (TLR) in the epithelial layer. These receptors act like security gate that get stimulated by what is in the gut environment. Between the cells are firm tight junctions, like tight connectors that keep the cells tightly fitted with one another. Underneath the epithelial layer is the lamina propria, a loose connective tissue that allows immune cells and inflammation markers to float through, preventing harmful substances from invading your body. Under this, is the blood supply.

Role of Toll-Like Receptors In SUDD

Toll-like receptors (TLRs) are like the body's security guards, helping to spot trouble in the gut. In symptomatic uncomplicated diverticular disease (SUDD), these guards become extra sensitive, especially around the diverticula.

Now, imagine these diverticula as little pockets in the colon wall. In SUDD, the tissue around these pockets changes, becoming more prone to inflammation. TLRs in these areas become more active, ready to react to any potential threats. When the TLR start getting more active, the tight junctions that hold the cells closely together become looser, thus allowing particles, allergens, irritants etc. to travel freely from the gut into the body itself.

As a result of these changes, the types of bacteria living around these diverticula can also change. Normally, our gut has a diverse community of bacteria, but in SUDD, this balance can shift. Some types of bacteria may thrive more in these altered areas, potentially worsening inflammation and symptoms like bloating, pain, and chronic inflammation.

For example, Barbara et al. (2010) found that TLRs are more active in people with SUDD compared to those without the condition, suggesting a role in symptom development.

Moreover, changes in gut bacteria composition can influence inflammation, as shown in a study by Colman et al. (2014). This supports the idea that alterations in bacteria types around diverticula could contribute to chronic inflammation in SUDD.

Understanding these connections helps us see how TLRs, changes in gut bacteria, and anatomical alterations around diverticula are linked to symptoms like bloating, pain, and chronic inflammation in SUDD.

Treatment Options

The Influence of Diet and Lifestyle on Toll-Like Receptor (TLR) Function in SUDD

In Symptomatic Uncomplicated Diverticular Disease (SUDD), diet and lifestyle significantly impact inflammation via modulation of Toll-Like Receptor (TLR) activity.

Dietary Fiber: A low-fiber diet alters gut microbiota, potentially triggering TLR activation and inflammation (Raskov et al., 2019). Increasing fiber intake supports microbial diversity and intestinal health.

Obesity: Obesity is linked to chronic low-grade inflammation and altered TLR function, elevating the risk for SUDD (Caviglia et al., 2017).

Physical Activity: Regular exercise can reduce inflammation and help regulate TLR activity (Humes et al., 2019).

Smoking: Smoking disrupts gut microbiota and promotes inflammation, influencing TLR activation (Tursi, 2016).

Antibiotics: Rifaximin reduces harmful bacteria and TLR4 activation, decreasing inflammation in SUDD (Tursi et al., 2016).

Sporebiotics: Sporebiotics, particularly *Bacillus subtilis*, *Bacillus clausii*, and *Bacillus coagulans* can modulate TLRs, reduce gut inflammation, and improve symptoms (Elshaghabee, F. M. F et al., 2017).

Prebiotics: Non-digestible fibers (e.g., in apples, onions, broccoli) feed beneficial bacteria and help regulate TLR function, supporting gut health (Barbara et al., 2019).

Practical Application

During Phase 2 of the diverticulitis low-roughage plan, consider adding a multi-strain Spore Forming Probiotic and prebiotic fibres to support microbial balance and reduce inflammation.

References

Barbara, G., et al. (2010). Toll-like receptor 2 and 4 expression in the intestinal mucosa of patients with symptomatic uncomplicated diverticular disease. BMC Gastroenterology, 10, 10. doi:10.1186/1471-230x-10-10

Barbara, G., Scaioli, E., Barbaro, M. R., Biagi, E., Laghi, L., Cremon, C., Corinaldesi, R. (2019). Gut microbiota, metabolome, and immune signatures in patients with uncomplicated diverticular disease. Gut, 68(6), 1083–1093. doi:10.1136/gutjnl-2018-316304

Caviglia, G. P., Rosso, C., Ribaldone, D. G., Dughera, F., Fagoonee, S., & Pellicano, R. (2017). The Role of Diet in the Pathogenesis of Colonic Diverticular Disease: Is There an Evidence-Based Relationship? Nutrients, 9(8), 805. doi:10.3390/nu9080805

Colman, R. J., et al. (2014). The commensal microbiota influences the susceptibility to colitis and colitis-associated colorectal cancer in IL-10-/- mice. Inflammatory Bowel Diseases, 20(12), 2319–2328. doi:10.1097/mib.0000000000000247

Elshaghabee, F. M. F., Rokana, N., Gulhane, R. D., Sharma, C., & Panwar, H. (2017). *Bacillus* as potential probiotics: Status, concerns, and future perspectives. *Frontiers in Microbiology, 8*, 1490. https://doi.org/10.3389/fmicb.2017.01490

Humes, D. J., Fleming, K. M., Spiller, R. C., & West, J. (2019). Concurrent drug use and the risk of perforated colonic diverticular disease: a population-based case-control study. Gut, 68(6), 1014–1020. doi:10.1136/gutjnl-2018-317829

Raskov, H., Burcharth, J., Pommergaard, H. C., & Rosenberg, J. (2019). Irritable bowel syndrome, the microbiota, and the gut-brain axis. Gut Microbes, 10(3), 224–236. doi:10.1080/19490976.2018.1515041

Tursi, A. (2016). Smoking in diverticular disease: A systematic review of the evidence. Colorectal Disease, 18(6), 528–539. doi:10.1111/codi.13307

Tursi, A., Brandimarte, G., Giorgetti, G. M., & Elisei, W. (2016). Assessment and grading of mucosal inflammation in colonic diverticular disease. Journal of Clinical Gastroenterology, 50(Suppl 1), S18–S22. doi:10.1097/mcg.0000000000000614

Chapter 9
Development of SIBO/IMO In Diverticular Disease

Small intestinal bacterial overgrowth (SIBO) and intestinal methanogen overgrowth (IMO) are conditions where there is an excess of bacteria, often from the colon, in the small intestine. This can happen in diverticular disease, where small pouches (diverticula) form in the colon wall.

How SIBO/IMO Can Develop In Diverticulitis

Diverticula Formation: Diverticula are like little pockets that form in the colon wall. They can trap food and bacteria, creating a breeding ground for bacterial overgrowth.

Altered Motility: In diverticular disease, the movement of the intestines can change. This can slow down the passage of food and bacteria, allowing them to accumulate and overgrow.

Stagnation of Contents: Food and bacteria can get stuck in the diverticula, creating stagnant areas where bacteria can thrive.

Bacterial Overgrowth: With the excess of bacteria in the colon, some can migrate backward into the small intestine or accumulate in the diverticula.

Fermentation: Once in the small intestine or diverticula, these bacteria ferment undigested carbohydrates, producing gases like hydrogen and methane. Methane-producing bacteria can also overgrow in the small intestine, leading to IMO.

Symptoms: SIBO/IMO can cause symptoms like bloating, abdominal discomfort, and changes in bowel habits, which are common in diverticular disease.

SIBO/IMO Treatment Options

Antibiotics

Antibiotics like Rifaximin can help by reducing the number of bacteria in the small intestine. This can improve symptoms and reduce bacterial fermentation. Refer to https://maximisednutrition.com/treatment-option-sibo-imo/ for more on this.

Sporebiotics: A New Ally in Gut Health and Diverticulitis Recovery

Unlike regular probiotics, **Sporebiotics** are a special type of beneficial bacteria that come with a tough outer shell. This natural "armour" helps them survive the journey through the stomach, where strong acids and bile can destroy most other probiotics. Thanks to this resilience, Sporebiotics make it all the way to the large intestine—exactly where diverticulitis happens—so they can start working right where they're needed most (Elshaghabee et al., 2017).

Some of the most well-studied Sporebiotics include *Bacillus subtilis*, *Bacillus clausii*, and *Bacillus coagulans*. These bacteria have powerful anti-inflammatory effects and help regulate the immune system. They've been shown to reduce inflammation in the gut and strengthen the gut lining, which often becomes weakened in people with diverticulitis (Tiwari & Shukla, 2017). One strain, *Bacillus coagulans*, may also help relieve symptoms like bloating and abdominal pain—especially helpful after a diverticulitis flare-up (Majeed et al., 2016).

Sporebiotics also play an important role in balancing the gut microbiome. They help keep harmful bacteria in check, support a healthy variety of gut microbes, and boost the production of short-chain fatty acids like **butyrate**—a substance that promotes healing and protects the colon (Pham et al., 2021).

Because of their strength, safety, and ability to target the large intestine, Sporebiotics are a promising addition to a holistic approach for managing diverticulitis. When used alongside a high-fiber diet, anti-inflammatory foods, and stress reduction techniques, they can support long-term gut health and recovery.

Read more on this blog post: https://maximisednutrition.com/spore-forming-probiotics-and-sibo/.

Dietary Modifications

Dietary changes can help manage SIBO/IMO. Avoiding fermentable carbohydrates that feed bacteria, known as the low FODMAP diet, may help reduce symptoms. Increasing fiber intake can also help by promoting regular bowel movements and preventing bacterial overgrowth.

Prokinetics

Prokinetic agents can improve intestinal motility, helping to move food and bacteria through the digestive tract more efficiently. This can reduce the risk of bacterial overgrowth and alleviate symptoms. Ginger is an example of a natural prokinetic.

If you have tried this four-stage dietary management plan for diverticulitis, and you still have symptoms of bloating, pain, etc., it may be that you have SIBO/IMO. Thus, a hydrogen methane breath test is recommended to see if you have SIBO/IMO. See articles on Hydrogen Methane Breath Tests on the website of Maximised Nutrition (maximisednutrition.com).

By addressing the underlying bacterial overgrowth and motility issues, these treatment options can help manage SIBO/IMO and improve symptoms in diverticular disease.

References

Elshaghabee, F. M. F., Rokana, N., Gulhane, R. D., Sharma, C., & Panwar, H. (2017). *Bacillus* as potential probiotics: Status, concerns, and future perspectives. *Frontiers in Microbiology, 8*, 1490. https://doi.org/10.3389/fmicb.2017.01490

Losurdo, G., et al. (2015). Probiotic monotherapy and Helicobacter pylori eradication: A systematic review with pooled-data analysis. World Journal of Gastroenterology, 21(10), 2512–2520. doi:10.3748/wjg.v21.i10.2512

Majeed, M., Nagabhushanam, K., Natarajan, S., Sivakumar, A., & Majeed, S. (2016). Evaluation of the probiotic *Bacillus coagulans* MTCC 5856 in the treatment of functional dyspepsia. *Indian Journal of Gastroenterology, 35*(6), 336–342.

Pham, L. N., Kanther, M., Semova, I., & Rawls, J. F. (2021). Interactions between commensal bacteria and the host immune system in health and disease. *Cell Host & Microbe, 17*(6), 692–703.

Pimentel, M., et al. (2006). Treatment of irritable bowel syndrome with rifaximin in clinical practice: A single center experience. Alimentary Pharmacology & Therapeutics, 24(4), 675–684. doi:10.1111/j.1365-2036.2006.03096.x

Rezaie, A., et al. (2017). Hydrogen and methane-based breath testing in gastrointestinal disorders: The North American consensus. The American Journal of Gastroenterology, 112(5), 775–784. doi:10.1038/ajg.2017.46

Chapter 10
Preventing Diverticulitis: Strategies and Tips

In this chapter, we will explore essential lifestyle and dietary changes that can help you maintain a healthy digestive system and avoid diverticular disease. Incorporating these strategies into your daily routine can improve your overall health and well-being while minimizing the risk of diverticulitis. Let us dive into these preventative measures and tips to help you lead a healthier, more comfortable life.

Preventative Measures

To reduce the risk of developing diverticula, consider the following preventative measures:

Vigorous Exercise

Engage in activities that make you sweat, such as running, cycling, swimming, or aerobic exercise. Regular vigorous exercise is beneficial for overall health and can help prevent diverticular disease. Exercise helps maintain a healthy weight, reduces inflammation, and promotes regular bowel movements, all of which are important for digestive health.

High-fiber diet

Consume 200 to 300 grams of fruits and vegetables daily, aiming for 9 servings to 11 servings each day. A serving is equivalent to the size of your hand when you are holding an object the size of an orange. A high-fiber diet helps maintain bowel health, prevents constipation, and promotes the growth of beneficial bacteria. Fiber adds bulk to the stool, making it easier to pass and reducing the pressure on the colon walls. Whole grains, nuts, seeds, and legumes are also excellent sources of fiber.

Since the start of diverticulitis may be due to an imbalance of gut microbiome, including green vegetables such as broccoli, spinach, kale, Swiss chard/Silverbeet, Bok choy etc. and as many colors of other fruit and vegetables provide a whole lot of prebiotic fibers that are foods to your gut bacteria. Thus, regular intake of green vegetable smoothies is also recommended. Always try to have one green vegetable with your dinner meals every night.

Vitamin D

Increase your vitamin D levels by spending 10 to 20 minutes in the sun each day, preferably in the morning or evening. Always protect your skin when exposed to the sun. Vitamin D plays a role in immune function and inflammation regulation. You can also get vitamin D from foods like fatty fish, fortified dairy products, and supplements.

Alcohol

The relationship between alcohol consumption and diverticular disease is still under investigation. It is best to consume alcohol in moderation and monitor its effects on your digestive health. Excessive alcohol intake can irritate the digestive tract and alter gut microbiota, increasing the risk of diverticular disease.

Dietary Tips

Avoid Nuts and High-Fiber Foods During Acute Episodes

If you experience an acute diverticulitis episode with bleeding or severe pain, avoid nuts and high-fiber foods to prevent irritation. During these times, a low-roughage diet can help reduce inflammation and allow the colon to heal.

Personalized Diet

Be aware of your symptoms and identify foods that cause discomfort. Some individuals may find that spicy foods or certain nuts exacerbate their symptoms. Keeping a food diary can help you track which foods trigger your symptoms and adjust your diet accordingly.

For most people, with no symptoms, in well stage, a Mediterranean diet option is suitable.

Variety and Balance

Maintain a balanced diet with a variety of foods. Avoid overly restrictive diets to ensure you receive adequate nutrition. Eating a diverse range of fruits, vegetables, grains, and proteins ensures you get all the essential nutrients your body needs for optimal health. The best dietary style to eat for healthy living is the Mediterranean Diet, which is a wholesome, high-fiber diet where protein sources are mainly from chicken, fish, lentils, legumes, chickpeas with some red meat, high in healthy fat, moderate in the amount of carbohydrate and protein.

Additional Preventative Strategies

Hydration

Drink plenty of water throughout the day. Staying hydrated helps your digestive system function smoothly and prevents constipation, which can exacerbate diverticular issues. Aim for at least 8 cups of water a day, more if you are active or live in a hot climate.

Regular Medical Check-Ups

Regular visits to your healthcare provider can help monitor your condition and make necessary adjustments to your diet and lifestyle. Early detection and management of potential issues can prevent complications.

Stress Management

Chronic stress can negatively affect your digestive health. Incorporate stress management techniques such as meditation/prayer, or deep breathing exercises into your daily routine. Finding healthy ways to manage stress can improve overall well-being and reduce the risk of digestive issues.

Social Engagement

Social engagement and social connectedness are key elements of positive health insofar as they reduce stress, improve mental well-being, and lower the risk of chronic diseases. Meaningful interactions not only enable individual resilience but also reinforce healthy behaviors, create emotional support networks, and lead to overall better health and longevity, enriching them with a feeling of belonging and purpose.

Regular Exercise

Regular exercise drastically cuts down on stress by prompting the release of endorphins, which are natural mood lifters and help with easing anxiety. It controls cortisol, a stress hormone in the body, in order to avoid chronic stress. Exercise promotes gut health through improvements in gut motility, reduced inflammation, and facilitating the growth of beneficial bacteria that may improve digestion and immunity. Exercise that requires oxygen, such as walking and cycling, was found to have beneficial effects on the gut microbiome through the increase in production of short-chain fatty acids that ensure the health and balance of the gut.

Probiotics & Prebiotics & Sporebiotics

Consider incorporating probiotics, sporebiotics and prebiotics into your diet through supplements or foods like yogurt, kefir, and fermented vegetables. Probiotics can help the existing beneficial bacteria to grow in the gut. Prebiotics (found in apple, chicory, dandelion greens, asparagus, and artichokes) feed the existing microbiome and help them to grow. A healthy gut microbiome supports digestion and can reduce inflammation.

Summary

Implementing these preventative measures and dietary tips can help reduce your risk of developing diverticula and manage diverticulitis effectively.

Be mindful of your body's responses to different foods and adjust your diet accordingly.

If you need personalized advice, especially for Australian and New Zealand clients, consider booking an online consultation for a discounted rate on my website: maximisednutrition.com.

Regular check-ups with your healthcare provider can also help manage your condition effectively.

Take care, stay healthy, and be proactive in managing diverticulitis. Incorporating these strategies into your daily routine can significantly improve your quality of life and reduce the risk of diverticular disease.

Chapter 11
21 Day Standard and Diabetic Menus and Shopping Lists

Standard Population

Week 1 Menu For Standard Population

Category	Monday	Tuesday	Wednesday	Thursday	Friday	Saturday	Sunday
	BREAKFAST						
Cereals	Rice Bubbles (Rice Krispies) OR Porridge with Sugar OR Cornflakes						
Dairy	Low Fat Milk OR Whole Milk OR Plain or Fruit Flavored yogurt						
	Peaches - Stewed	Pears - Stewed	Apples - Stewed	Pears - Stewed	Peaches - Stewed	Apples - Stewed	Peaches - Stewed
	Fruit Juice						
Breads	White Toast OR White Bread OR Whole Meal Bread						
Spreads	Margarine or Butter or Avocado Spread With Honey OR Peanut Butter (Smooth) OR Apricot Jam Nutritional Yeast for Extra B Vitamins						
	Clear Fruit Juice						
	Morning Tea (choose 1 option)						
Morning Tea	Plain Crackers & Cheese	Plain Crackers & Cheese	Plain Cracker, Cottage Cheese	Plain Cracker, Cottage Cheese	Plain Crackers and Cream Cheese	Plain Crackers & Cheese	Plain Natural yogurt
	OR Plain Biscuits						
	LUNCH						
Soup	Cream of Pumpkin	Crème of Tomato	Crème of Tomato	Cream of Chicken	Crème of Tomato	Cream of Pumpkin	Crème of Tomato
	Sandwich (made with white or wholemeal bread)						
Sandwich	Ham	Egg	Beef	Ham	Chicken	Corned Silverside	Cheese
	Extra						
Bakery	White Bread OR Rice Wafer OR Wholemeal Bread						
Spreads	Butter or Margarine or Avocado Spread With Peanut Butter (smooth) OR Apricot Jam						
	Fresh Fruit *Soft Banana*						
	Afternoon Tea (choose 1 option)						
Afternoon Tea	Plain Crackers Cottage Cheese	Plain Crackers & Cream Cheese	Plain yogurt	Plain yogurt	Plain Crackers & Cheese	Plain Crackers and Cream Cheese	Plain Crackers & Cheese
	OR Plain Biscuits or Banana						
	DINNER						
	Citrus Salmon, Pea Puree, Mashed Sweet Potato	Beef Burger	Apricot Chicken with Steamed Rice	Creamy Prawn Pasta	Braised Lamb Chop with Rice	Beef Meatball in Tortilla Wrap with Carrot, Cucumber,	Roast Pork, Mashed Potato, Boiled Pumpkin Swiss Chard / Silverbeet
	Salt AND/OR Pepper						
	Dessert (choose maximum of 2 Options)						
	Custard or Ice Cream (plain) with Jelly						
	Pears - Stewed	Peaches - Stewed	Pears - Stewed	Peaches - Stewed	Apples - Stewed with Cinnamon	Pears - Stewed	Apples - Stewed with Cinnamon
	Supper (choose 1 option)						
Supper	Plain Crackers, Cottage Cheese	Fruit Flavored yogurt	Plain Crackers & Cheese	Plain Crackers & Cheese	Fruit Flavored yogurt	Fruit Flavored yogurt	Plain Crackers & Cream Cheese
	Or Plain Biscuit with A Hot Milky Cocoa Drink						

For Morning Tea, Afternoon Tea, Supper, a hot chocolate option is recommended at times

Week 2 Menu for Standard Population

Category	Monday	Tuesday	Wednesday	Thursday	Friday	Saturday	Sunday
	BREAKFAST						
Cereals	Rice Bubbles (Rice Krispies) OR Porridge with Sugar OR Cornflakes						
Dairy	Low Fat Milk OR Whole Milk OR Plain OR Fruit flavored yogurt						
	Pears - Stewed	Apples - Stewed	Peaches - Stewed	Apples - Stewed	Peaches - Stewed	Apples - Stewed	Pears - Stewed
	Fruit Juice						
Breads	White Toast OR White Bread OR Whole meal Bread (no seeds or broken grains)						
Spreads	Margarine or Butter or Avocado Spread with Honey OR Peanut Butter (Smooth) OR Apricot Jam Nutritional Yeast for Extra Vitamin Bs						
	Morning Tea (choose 1 option)						
	Plain Crackers & Cheese						
	OR Plain Biscuits	Plain Crackers & Cheese	Plain Crackers, Cottage Cheese	Plain Crackers, Cottage Cheese	Plain Crackers & Cream Cheese	Plain Crackers & Cheese	Plain Natural yogurt
	LUNCH						
Soup	Crème of Chicken	Crème of Tomato	Cream of Pumpkin	Cream of Chicken	Crème of Tomato	Cream of Pumpkin	Cream of Chicken
	Sandwich (made with white or wholemeal bread)						
Sandwich	Ham	Tuna	Ham	Corned Silverside	Cheese	Ham	Cheese
	White Bread OR Rice Wafer OR Wholemeal Bread						
Bakery	Margarine or Avocado or Butter with Honey OR Peanut Butter (Smooth) OR Apricot Jam						
	Fresh Fruit (soft banana)						
Fresh Fruit	***Afternoon Tea***						
	Plain Biscuits	Plain Crackers, Cream Cheese	Plain yogurt	Plain Crackers Cheese	Plain yogurt	Plain Crackers Cottage Cheese	Plain Crackers & Cream Cheese
	DINNER						
Main	Scotch Fillet, Mashed Potato Steamed Pumpkin and Broccoli	Bacon Egg Potato Top Pi	Moroccan Lamb Shank, Sweet Potato / Kumara, Cucumber, Carrot	Pan Fried Fish with Lemon Slice, Mashed Potato, Cauliflower, Broccoli	Chicken in Basil Sauce	Spaghetti Bolognaise with Broccoli	Corned Silverside Mashed Potato, Beetroot, Swiss Chard / Silverbeet
Condiments	Salt /Pepper						
	Dessert						
	Custard Or Plain Ice Cream with Jelly						
	Peaches - Stewed	Pears - Stewed	Apples - Stewed with Cinnamon	Peaches - Stewed	Pears - Stewed	Peaches - Stewed	Apples - Stewed with Cinnamon
	Supper						
Supper	OR Plain Biscuit with Hot Milky Cocoa Drink	Fruit Flavored yogurt	Plain Crackers & Cheese	Fruit Flavored yogurt	Plain Crackers & Cheese	Fruit Flavored yogurt	Plain Crackers & Cheese

For Morning Tea, Afternoon Tea, Supper, a hot chocolate option is recommended at times

Week 3 Menu for Standard Population

Category	Monday	Tuesday	Wednesday	Thursday	Friday	Saturday	Sunday
	BREAKFAST						
Cereals	Rice Bubbles (Rice Krispies) OR Porridge with Sugar OR Cornflakes						
Sugar	Sugar						
	Pears - Stewed	Apples - Stewed	Peaches - Stewed	Apples - Stewed	Peaches - Stewed	Apples - Stewed	Pears - Stewed
	Fruit Juice						
Breads	White Toast OR White Bread OR Whole meal Bread (no seeds or broken grains)						
Spreads	Margarine or Butter or Avocado Spread with Honey OR Peanut Butter (Smooth) OR Apricot Jam						
	Nutritional Yeast for Extra Vitamin Bs						
	Morning Tea (choose 1 option)						
Morning Tea	Plain Crackers & Cheese	Plain Crackers & Cheese	Plain Crackers, Cottage Cheese	Plain Crackers, Cottage Cheese	Plain Crackers & Cream Cheese	Plain Crackers & Cheese	Plain Natural yogurt
	OR Plain Biscuits						
	LUNCH						
Soup	Cream of Pumpkin	Crème of Tomato	Cream of Pumpkin	Cream of Chicken	Crème of Tomato	Cream of Pumpkin	Cream of Chicken
	Sandwich (made with white or wholemeal bread)						
Sandwich	Cheese	Tuna	Ham	Corned Beef Silverside	Cheese	Ham	Cheese
	Extra						
Bakery	White Bread OR Rice Wafer Or Wholemeal bread						
Spreads	Margarine or Avocado or Butter with Honey OR Peanut Butter (Smooth) OR Apricot Jam						
	Fresh Fruit (soft banana)						
	Afternoon Tea (choose 1 option)						
	Plain yogurt	Plain Crackers, Cream Cheese	Plain yogurt	Plain Crackers Cheese	Plain yogurt	Plain Crackers Cottage Cheese	Plain Crackers & Cream Cheese
	OR Plain Biscuits						
	DINNER						
	Beef Curry with Rice and Spinach	Marinated Pork in Pita Bread	Chicken Chow Mein	Beef Casserole with Steamed Rice	Baked Fish in Coconut Cream with Mashed Potato, Spinach, Carrot	Silverbeet (Swiss Chard) Lamb Lasagna	Chicken Meatballs with Rice, Broccoli, Cauliflower & Parsley Sauce
Condiments	Salt AND/OR Pepper						
Dessert	***Dessert***						
	Custard Or Plain Ice Cream With Jelly						
	Peaches - Stewed	Pears - Stewed	Apples - Stewed with Cinnamon	Peaches - Stewed	Pears - Stewed	Peaches - Stewed	Apples - Stewed with Cinnamon
	Supper (choose 1 option)						
Supper	Plain Crackers & Cheese	Plain yogurt	Plain Crackers & Cheese	Plain yogurt	Plain Crackers & Cheese	Plain yogurt	Plain Crackers & Cheese
	OR Plain Biscuit with Hot Milky Cocoa Drink						

For Morning Tea, Afternoon Tea, Supper, a hot chocolate option is recommended at times

Diabetic Population

Week 1 Menu for Diabetic Population

Category	Monday	Tuesday	Wednesday	Thursday	Friday	Saturday	Sunday
	BREAKFAST						
Cereals	Rice Bubbles (Rice Krispies) OR Porridge with Artificial Sweetener OR Cornflakes						
Dairy	Low Fat Milk OR Whole Milk OR Plain yogurt						
	Peaches – Stewed (drained)	Pears – Stewed (drained)	Apples – Stewed (drained)	Pears – Stewed (drained)	Peaches – Stewed (drained)	Apples – Stewed (drained)	Peaches – Stewed (drained)
	Cordial – sugar free						
Breads	White Toast OR White Bread OR Whole Meal Bread						
Spreads	Margarine or Butter or Avocado Spread with Peanut Butter (smooth) OR Diabetic Jam						
	Nutritional Yeast for Extra Vitamin Bs						
	Morning Tea (choose 1 option)						
Morning Tea	Plain Crackers & Cheese	Plain Crackers & Cheese	Plain crackers, cottage cheese	Plain Crackers, Cottage Cheese	Plain Crackers & Cream Cheese	Plain Crackers & Cheese	Plain Crackers, Tuna
	OR Plain Biscuits or digestive with glass of milk						
LUNCH	**LUNCH**						
Soup	Cream of Pumpkin	Crème of Tomato	Crème of Tomato	Cream of Chicken	Crème of Tomato	Cream of Pumpkin	Crème of Tomato
	Sandwich (made with white or whole meal bread)						
Sandwich	Ham	Egg	Beef	Ham	Chicken	Corned Silverside	Cheese
	Extra						
Bakery	White Bread OR Wholemeal Bread OR Rice Wafer						
Spreads	Margarine or Avocado or Butter with Peanut Butter (smooth) OR Diabetic Jam						
Fresh Fruit	Allowed Fruit						
	Afternoon Tea (choose 1 option)						
Afternoon Tea	Plain Crackers Cottage Cheese	Plain Crackers & Cream Cheese	Plain yogurt	Plain yogurt	Plain Crackers, & Cheese	Plain Crackers and Cream Cheese	Plain Crackers, & Cheese
	OR Plain Biscuits with glass of milk						
DINNER	**DINNER**						
	Citrus Salmon with Pea Puree with Mashed Sweet Potato /Kumara	Beef Burger	Apricot Chicken with Steamed Rice	Creamy Prawn Pasta	Braised Lamb Chop with Rice	Beef Meatball in Tortilla Wrap with Cucumber, Carrot	Roast Pork, Mashed Potato, Pumpkin Swiss Chard / Silverbeet
Condiments	S/alt AND/OR Pepper						
Dessert	***Dessert (choose maximum of 2 Options)***						
	Custard (sugar free) with Diabetic Jelly						
	Pears – Stewed (drained)	Peaches – Stewed (drained)	Pears – Stewed (drained)	Peaches – Stewed (drained)	Apples - Stewed with Cinnamon (drained)	Pears – Stewed (drained)	Apples - Stewed with Cinnamon (drained)
Supper	***Supper***						
Supper	Plain Crackers, Cottage Cheese	Plain Crackers, Tuna	Plain Crackers & Cream Cheese	Plain Crackers, Tuna	Plain Crackers, Tuna	Plain Crackers & Cream Cheese	Plain Crackers, Tuna
	With a glass of milk						

If needed for blood sugar control over night, can have a protein sandwich made with white bread for supper.

Week 2 Menu for Diabetic Population

Category	Monday	Tuesday	Wednesday	Thursday	Friday	Saturday	Sunday
	BREAKFAST						
Cereals	Rice Bubbles (Rice Krispies) OR Porridge with Artificial Sweetener OR Cornflakes						
Dairy	Low Fat Milk OR Whole Milk OR Plain yogurt						
	Pears – Stewed (drained)	Apples – Stewed (drained)	Peaches – Stewed (drained)	Apples – Stewed (drained)	Peaches – Stewed (drained)	Apples – Stewed (drained)	Pears – Stewed (drained)
	Cordial – sugar free						
Breads	White Toast OR White Bread OR WHOLEMEAL BREAD (no seeds or broken grains)						
Spreads	Margarine or Butter or Avocado Spread with Peanut Butter (smooth) OR Diabetic Jam						
	Morning Tea (choose 1 option)						
	Plain Crackers, & Cheese	Plain Crackers, Cheese	Plain Crackers, Cottage Cheese	Plain Crackers, Cottage Cheese	Plain Crackers & Cream Cheese	Plain Crackers & Cheese	Plain Natural yogurt
	OR Plain or Digestive Biscuits with Glass of Milk						
	LUNCH						
Soup	Cream of Pumpkin	Crème of Tomato	Cream of Pumpkin	Cream of Chicken	Crème of Tomato	Cream of Pumpkin	Cream of Chicken
	Sandwich (made with white or wholemeal bread)						
Sandwich	Cheese	Tuna	Ham	Salmon	Cheese	Ham	Cheese
	Extra						
Bakery	White Bread OR Wholemeal Bread OR Rice Wafer						
Spreads	Plant Based Spread or Avocado or Butter with Peanut Butter (smooth) OR Diabetic Jam						
Fresh Fruit	Allowed Fruit						
	Afternoon Tea (choose 1 option)						
	Plain yogurt	Plain Crackers, Cream Cheese	Plain yogurt	Plain Crackers, Cheese	Plain yogurt	Plain Crackers Cottage Cheese	Plain Crackers & Cream Cheese
	OR Plain or Digestive Biscuits with Milk						
	DINNER						
	Scotch Fillet, Mashed Potato, Steamed Pumpkin & Broccoli	Bacon Egg Potato Top Pie	Moroccan Lamb Shank, Sweet Potato (Kumara), Cucumber, Carrot	Pan Fried Fish with Lemon Slice, Mashed Potato, Cauliflower, Broccoli	Chicken in Basil Sauce	Spaghetti Bolognaise with Broccoli	Corned Silverside, Mashed Potato, Beetroot, Swiss Chard (Silverbeet)
Condiments	Salt AND/OR Pepper						
Dessert	**Dessert**						
	Custard – Sugar Free with Diabetic Jelly						
	Peaches – Stewed (drained)	Pears – Stewed (drained)	Apples - Stewed with Cinnamon (drained)	Peaches – Stewed (drained)	Pears – Stewed (drained)	Peaches – Stewed (drained)	Apples - Stewed with Cinnamon (drained)
Supper	**Supper**						
Supper	Plain Crackers & Cream Cheese	Plain Crackers, Tuna	Plain Crackers & Cream Cheese	Plain Crackers, Tuna	Plain Crackers, Tuna	Plain Crackers, Cottage Cheese	Plain Crackers, Tuna
	with a glass of milk						

If needed for blood sugar control over night, can have a protein sandwich made with white bread for supper.

Week 3 Menu for Diabetic Population

Category	Monday	Tuesday	Wednesday	Thursday	Friday	Saturday	Sunday
	BREAKFAST						
Cereals	Rice Bubbles (Rice Krispies) OR Porridge with Artificial Sweetener OR Cornflakes						
Dairy	Low Fat Milk OR Whole Milk OR Plain yogurt						
	Peaches – Stewed (drained)	Pears – Stewed (drained)	Apples – Stewed (drained)	Pears – Stewed (drained)	Peaches - Stewed (drained)	Apples – Stewed (drained)	Peaches – Stewed (drained)
	Cordial – sugar free						
Breads	White Toast OR White Bread OR Wholemeal Bread						
Spreads	Margarine or Butter with Peanut Butter (smooth) OR Diabetic Jam						
	Morning tea (choose 1 option)						
	Plain Crackers & Cheese	Plain Crackers & Cheese	Plain crackers, cottage cheese	Plain crackers, cottage cheese	Plain Crackers and Cream Cheese	Plain Crackers & Cheese	Plain yogurt
	OR Plain or Digestive Biscuits (Graham Crackers) with Glass of Milk						
	LUNCH						
Soup	crème of tomato	Cream of Chicken	crème of tomato	Cream of Pumpkin	crème of tomato	Cream of Pumpkin	crème of tomato
	Sandwich (made with white or Wholemeal bread)						
Sandwich	Ham	Egg	Salmon	Ham	Beef	Ham	Egg
Extra	***Extra***						
Bakery	White Bread OR Wholemeal OR Rice Wafer						
Spreads	Margarine or Butter with Peanut Butter (smooth) OR Diabetic Jam						
Fresh Fruit	Allowed Fruit						
	Afternoon tea (choose 1 option)						
	plain yogurt	Plain Crackers, Cream Cheese	plain yogurt	Plain Crackers, Cream Cheese	plain yogurt	Plain Crackers Cottage Cheese	Plain Crackers & Cheese
	OR Plain or Digestive Biscuits (Graham Crackers) with Milk						
	DINNER						
	Beef Curry with Rice and Spinach	Marinated Pork in Pita Bread	Chicken Chow Mein	Beef Casserole with Steamed Rice	Baked Fish in Coconut Cream with Mashed Potato, Spinach, Carrot	Silverbeet (Swiss Chard) Lamb Lasagna	Chicken Meatballs with Rice, Broccoli, Cauliflower & Parsley Sauce
Dessert	***Dessert (choose maximum of 2 Options)***						
	Custard (Sugar Free) with Diabetic Jelly						
	Pears – Stewed (drained)	Peaches – Stewed (drained)	Pears – Stewed (drained)	Peaches – Stewed (drained)	Apples - Stewed with Cinnamon (drained)	Pears – Stewed (drained)	Apples - Stewed with Cinnamon (drained)
	Supper						
Supper	plain Crackers & cream cheese	plain crackers, margarine, tuna	plain crackers, cottage cheese	plain crackers, margarine, tuna	plain crackers, cottage cheese	plain crackers, margarine, tuna	Plain Crackers & cream cheese
	with a glass of milk						

If needed for blood sugar control over night, can have a protein sandwich made with white bread for supper.

Shopping Lists

Shopping List - Week 1

Pantry Items ☐ Breadcrumbs ☐ Cornflour ☐ Flour ☐ Custard Powder ☐ Peanut Butter -smooth ☐ Nutmeg – ground ☐ Paprika - ground ☐ Rosemary – dried ☐ Black Pepper – ground ☐ Cumin – ground ☐ Salt ☐ Pepper – ground, black ☐ Pepper – ground, white ☐ Italian Herb Mix ☐ Hot drink options: tea, coffee, drinking chocolate etc.	☐ Tomato Sauce ☐ Worcestershire Sauce ☐ Ready made bolognaise sauce ☐ Tomato Paste ☐ Mayonnaise ☐ Garlic – to make garlic infused oil ☐ Onion – to make onion infused oil ☐ Honey ☐ Jam (or low sugar option) ☐ Sugar (not for those with diabetes) ☐ Clear Juice (apple, pear or orange) or get greens to make own green juices (see recipe section) ☐ Sugar free / Low sugar clear juice ☐ Olive Oil 2 Litres ☐ Margarine / butter A tub ☐ Nutritional Yeast ☐ Diabetic Jelly (for diabetics)

Dairy / Eggs		*Fruit & Vegetables*	
☐ Milk	2 L/1.2 gal	☐ Apricots, can, quartered	100g/3oz
☐ Get extra milk for smoothies		☐ Peaches – can, stewed	3 cans
☐ Egg	1 dozen	☐ Pears – can, stewed	3 cans
☐ Cheese (plain)	a block	☐ Apples – can, stewed	3 cans
☐ Cottage Cheese	1 x 250g/8oz	☐ Banana (not for those with diabetes)	3-4
☐ Cream Cheese	1 x 250g/8oz	☐ Avocado	3 medium
☐ Plain Yogurt	500g/18.8oz	☐ Beetroot - canned	
☐ Ice-cream (for standard menu)		☐ Broccoli	½ head
☐ Get extra yogurt for smoothies as needed.		☐ Carrot	2 medium
Rice & Cereals		☐ Cucumber	1
☐ Linguine Pasta	170g/6oz	☐ Lemon	3
☐ Rice	2 cups	☐ Frozen Peas	1 cup
☐ Tortilla Wrap	4	☐ Potato	1 medium
☐ Cornflakes		☐ Pumpkin	100g/3.5oz
☐ Fine Rolled Oats		☐ Silverbeet	100g/3.5oz
☐ Rice Bubbles / Ricies/Rice Krispies		☐ Sweet Potato / Kumara	1 medium
☐ Bread (white/wholemeal)	1-2 loaf/sliced	☐ —	
☐ Plain crackers	2x packets	☐ Get extra fruit/vegetables for the green juices / smoothies as needed	
☐ Rice Waters	1 packet		
☐ Plain Biscuit or low sugar biscuit / Digestive Biscuits (Graham Crackers) (for diabetes)	1 pack		

Shopping List - Week 1 Continued

Seafood & Meats	***To make home made soup***
☐ Beef Mince 2 x 200g/7oz ☐ Burger Buns 2 ☐ Diced boneless chicken 200g/7oz ☐ Lamb Loin chips 230g /½ lb ☐ Pork Shoulder Roast 200g/7oz ☐ Prawn – shelled 280g/10oz ☐ Salmon steak 200g/7oz ☐ Canned Tuna / Salmon 1 can (for those with Diabetes) ☐ Ham – shaved 60g/2oz for 1 servings of or 120g/4oz for 2 servings ☐ Chicken Deli cooked 60g/2oz for 1 servings of or 120g/4oz for 2 servings ☐ Beef sliced – Deli cooked 60g/2oz for 1 servings of or 120g/4oz for 2 servings	<u>Crème of Chicken Soup</u> ☐ Diced Chicken 340g/¾ lb ☐ Parsley 1 large bunch ☐ Carrot 2 large ☐ Potato 1 large ☐ Chicken Broth 1 cup ☐ Cream or Coconut Cream ½ cup <u>Cream of Pumpkin Soup</u> ☐ Pumpkin 1 whole ☐ Chicken or Vegetable Broth 1.5 L (3 x 4.5 oz packets) ☐ Cream 500ml/14.5oz <u>Cream of Tomato</u> ☐ Canned diced tomato 1 can ☐ Chicken or Vegetable Broth 1 cup

Shopping List - Week 2

Pantry Items

- ☐ Bay leaves 1
- ☐ Cloves 4
- ☐ Coriander Powder
- ☐ Turmeric powder
- ☐ Dried Basil
- ☐ Paprika Powder
- ☐ Cornflour
- ☐ Flour
- ☐ Mustard Sauce (seedless)
- ☐ Diabetic Jelly
- ☐ Ice Cream (for standard population)

Fruit & Vegetables

- ☐ Avocado 3
- ☐ Broccoli 1
- ☐ Potato 4-6 medium
- ☐ Pumpkin 1 large
- ☐ Carrot 2 medium
- ☐ Sweet Potato / Kumara 2 medium
- ☐ Swiss Chard / Silverbeet 8 oz
- ☐ Lemon 1
- ☐ Get extra fruit/vegetables for green juices and smoothies as needed.

Seafood & Meat

- ☐ Beef Mince 220g/8oz
- ☐ Corned Beef / Silverside 250g/9oz
- ☐ Diced Chicken 220g/8oz
- ☐ Diced Shoulder Bacon (rind removed): 200g/7oz
- ☐ Lamb Shank 2 shanks
- ☐ Scotch Fillet 240g/8oz
- ☐ Fish Fillet 2 Fillet (1 fillet = 120g/4oz)

Dairy / Eggs

- ☐ Cheese - grated
- ☐ Milk 2L/1/2 Gal
- ☐ Eggs ½ dozen
- ☐ yogurt 500g/18.8oz

Rice & Cereals

- ☐ Dried Spaghetti 120g/4oz

Check from last week if you need more of the following:

☐ Cornflakes ☐ Fine Rolled Oats ☐ Rice Bubbles / Ricies / Rice Krispies ☐ Bread (white, wholemeal) 1 -2 loaf / sliced ☐ Plain crackers 2 x packets	☐ Margarine ☐ Butter ☐ Ham sliced 60g/2oz ☐ Rice Waters 1 packet ☐ Plain Biscuit or low sugar biscuit / Digestive Biscuits (Graham Crackers) (for diabetes) 1 packet
To make home made soup <u>Crème of Chicken Soup</u> ☐ Diced Chicken 340g / ¾ lb ☐ Parsley 1 large bunch ☐ Carrot 2 large ☐ Potato 1 large ☐ Chicken Broth 1 cup ☐ Cream or Coconut Cream ½ cup <u>Cream of Pumpkin Soup</u> ☐ Pumpkin 1 whole ☐ Chicken or Vegetable Broth 1.5 L (3 x 4.5 oz packets) ☐ Cream 500ml/14.5oz <u>Cream of Tomato</u> ☐ Canned diced tomato 1 can ☐ Chicken or Vegetable Broth 1 cup	☐ Apricots, can, quartered 100g/3oz ☐ Peaches – can, stewed 3 cans ☐ Pears – can, stewed 3 cans ☐ Apples – can, stewed 3 cans ☐ Banana 3-4 medium (not for those with diabetes)

Shopping List - Week 3

Pantry Items

- ☐ Cardamon Pods 2
- ☐ Cinnamon Stick 3cm long
- ☐ Coriandar seeds 2 Tb
- ☐ Dried Basil Leaves
- ☐ Fennel seed, ground
- ☐ Fennel seed 1 tsp
- ☐ Ginger powder
- ☐ Star Anise 1 flower
- ☐ Coconut Cream 200g/7oz
- ☐ Diabetic Jelly
- ☐ Honey
- ☐ Oyster Sauce
- ☐ Sesane oil
- ☐ Soy sauce
- ☐ Tomato Pasata Sauce (strained pureed tomato) 250g /8.8oz
- ☐ Kebab skewers 4
- ☐ Ice cream (for standard menu)
- ☐ Custard powder

Fruit & Vegetables

- ☐ Avocado 3
- ☐ Broccoli 1
- ☐ Beetroot - sliced 1 can
- ☐ Carrot 8 medium
- ☐ Cauliflower ½ head
- ☐ Lemon 1
- ☐ Onion 1
- ☐ Potato 3 medium
- ☐ Swiss Chard / Silverbeet 8 leaves
- ☐ Baby Spinach 500g/18oz 5 cups
- ☐ Sweet potato / kumara 1 medium

Rice & Cereals

- ☐ Chow Mein Noodles 85g/3 oz
- ☐ Fresh Lasagna sheets 3 sheets
- ☐ Pita Bread 2 (6inch)
- ☐ Rice (basmati) 500g/18oz

Seafood & Meat	Dairy & Egg
☐ Beef strips or diced 220g/½ lb ☐ Beef diced 220g/½ lb ☐ Chicken drumsticks 4 ☐ Chicken Tenderloin or thighs 200g /6oz ☐ Fish Fillet 200g/7oz) or 2 fillets ☐ Lamb Mince 200g /7oz ☐ Pork sirloin 220g/½ lb	☐ Cheese ☐ Milk 2L/1/2 gal ☐ Egg ½ dozen

Check from last week if you need more of the following:

☐ Cornflakes ☐ Fine Rolled Oats ☐ Rice Bubbles / Ricies/Rice Krispies ☐ Bread (white, wholemeal) 1-2 loaf / sliced ☐ Plain crackers 2 x packets	☐ Margarine ☐ Butter ☐ Ham sliced: 60g/2oz or 120g/4oz ☐ Rice Waters 1 packet ☐ Plain Biscuit or low sugar biscuit / Digestive Biscuits (Graham Crackers) (for diabetes) 1 packet
To make home made soup <u>Crème of Chicken Soup</u> ☐ Diced Chicken 340g / ¾ Ib ☐ Parsley 1 large bunch ☐ Carrot 2 large ☐ Potato 1 large ☐ Chicken Broth 1 cup ☐ Cream or Coconut Cream ½ cup <u>Cream of Pumpkin Soup</u> ☐ Pumpkin 1 whole ☐ Chicken or Vegetable Broth 1.5 L (3 x 4.5 oz packets) ☐ Cream 500ml/14.5oz <u>Cream of Tomato</u> ☐ Canned diced tomato 1 can ☐ Chicken or Vegetable Broth 1 cup	☐ Apricots, can, quartered 100g/3oz ☐ Peaches – can, stewed 3 cans ☐ Pears – can, stewed 3 cans ☐ Apples – can, stewed 3 cans ☐ Banana 3-4 medium (not for those with diabetes)

Chapter 12
Recipes

Fruit Juice Recipes

(Including Green Juice)

Clear fruit juices especially those freshly juiced provide gut healing nutrients such as polyphenols that can help in preventing inflammation. They can also help provide those extra nutrients for the good microbiome, helping to maintain a healthy microbiome balance.

Just note that for clear fluid diet, free fluid diet and low roughage diet, these juices must not have any pulps. As you transition to a high fiber diet, you can easily convert these recipes into a smoothie which includes the fiber components. Your good gut bugs love these fibers.

You can add herbs and spices to these juices when appropriate. Turmeric, basil, mint, sage, oregano, rosemary etc. all have anti-bacterial, anti-inflammatory functions. Below are just some simple examples.

You can use apple or pineapple as the juice base and build your flavors from there on. Be daring.

Note, though, if you have burping or reflux, you may have SIBO (small bacterial intestinal overgrowth) or intestinal dysbiosis (wrong bugs growing in the wrong area of your gut). In that case, I suggest to either reduce the amount you are having or not have the specific juices that use fruit.

If you have diabetes, then watch for the sugar levels. Some of these juices may not be ideal for you (those using apple, pineapple, orange juice or beetroot for example).

These recipes are for one (1) serving.

Dandelion, Spinach, Cucumber, Celery Juice

Dandelion leaves -	6 - 8 leaves
Spinach leaves - chopped	½ cup
Cucumber - diced	1
Celery	4-6 stalk
Ginger - chopped	1 inch

Wash all your vegetables before juicing. Juice all ingredients together.

Spinach, Cucumber, Carrot, Green Apple Juice

Baby Spinach - chopped	1 cup
Green Grapes	20
Cucumber - diced	1
Carrot- scrabbed, chopped	1 medium
Granny Smith Apple - chopped	1
Green Pepper (optional) for zing!	½ (deseeded).

Wash all of these before chopping. Juice.

Celery, Broccoli, Orange, Cucumber Juice

Celery	4 stalks
Broccoli - florets	¼ broccoli
Orange	2
Cucumber	1

Wash, dice, chop, and juice!

Watermelon, Mint, Spinach Juice

Mint leaves	6 -8 depending on your taste
Watermelon	1 cup- chopped
Baby Spinach	½ cup

Wash mint leaves, and baby spinach leaves. Chop them. Add all the ingredients to the juicer and juice.

Basil, Coconut Water, Strawberry, Carrot Juice

Basil leaves - chopped	½ Tb
Coconut Water	1 cup
Strawberry - frozen	½ cup
Carrot - scrubbed and chopped	1 medium

Add all the ingredients to juicer, juice and drink.

Apple, Celery, Parsley, Ginger Juice

Apple	2
Celery	6 sticks
Parsley	1 bunch
Ginger	½ inch

Wash and dice apples, parsley, celery, and ginger. Add in juicer. Juice and drink.

Smoothie Recipes

Smoothies are a great way to get some nutrients in. Adding a protein powder to these smoothies can help in getting the needed protein into your diet.

If a smoothie is a meal replacement, aim to have around 25g to 30g of protein in a serving.

You can use three of these options to increase the protein amounts in your smoothie:

- Use of a Protein powder: this can be whey protein based or plant protein based (like pea protein isolate).
- Use of skim milk powder
- Use of Greek Yogurt or yogurt higher in protein. Use a low fat, low sugar option.

If you have diarrhea or sore tummy, you can replace the yogurt/milk with dairy free milk or yogurt but add in the pea protein isolate. It may be that your lactase enzyme (that breaks down cow's milk sugar lactose) is low due to infection / inflammation so going dairy free can help.

Note that these smoothies need to have minimum insoluble fiber for phase 2 of the plan. In the transition phase, you can blitz the smoothie into a smooth puree texture, keeping some of the fiber and in phase 4, you can add fiber. Though I caution against using small unbroken seeds or corn even in phase 4.

Also note, banana skin is a great prebiotic (food to grow probiotic bugs in our tummy) so in phase 3 and 4, you can add the banana skin (chop the ends of the banana) and rinse the outside of the skin with hot water and then add to the smoothie.

Banana Pineapple Smoothie

Ingredients	**Quantity**	**Method**
Greek yogurt - low fat, low sugar	170g or 6oz	Put all in a jug or nutri-bullet and biltz. Pour into a glass and drink!
Banana - Ripe	1 medium	
Pineapple Juice	1 cup	
Skim Milk Powder	2 Tb	

Nutritional Analysis Per Serving

USA: Energy (kj/kcal): 1479 (353), Protein (g): 25, Carbohydrate (g): 60, Sugar (g): 54, Total Fat (g): 1.5, Sodium (mg): 88 Dietary Fiber (g): 3.5

Australia: Energy (kj/kcal): 1507 (360), Protein (g): 23, Carbohydrate (g): 60, Sugar (g): 53, Total Fat (g): 0.9, Sodium (mg): 88 Dietary Fiber (g): 2.1

New Zealand: Energy (kj/kcal): 1905 (455), Protein (g): 24, Carbohydrate (g): 70, Sugar (g): 64, Total Fat (g): 8.3, Sodium (mg): 155, Dietary Fiber (g): 2.6

Mocha Smoothie

Ingredients	**Quantity**	**Method**
Milk, standard - cold	1 Cup	Put all in a jug or nutri-bullet and biltz. Pour into a glass and drink!
Coffee - instant	1 tsp (may want more!)	
Skim milk powder or protein powder	2 Tb	
Cocoa Powder	1 Tb (may want more)	

Nutritional Analysis Per Serving

USA: Energy (kj/kcal): 1207 (288) Protein (g): 25, Carbohydrate (g): 14, Sugar (g): 15, Total Fat (g): 15 Sodium (mg): 210, Dietary Fiber (g): 7.7

Australia: Energy (kj/kcal): 1283 (307) Protein (g): 21, Carbohydrate (g): 33, Sugar (g): 10, Total Fat (g): 6.5, Sodium (mg): 223, Dietary Fiber (g): 2.3

New Zealand: Energy (kj/kcal): 1328 (317), Protein (g): 27, Carbohydrate (g): 16.5, Sugar (g): 12.5, Total Fat (g): 16, Sodium (mg): 124, Dietary Fiber (g): 2.3

Peanut Butter Smoothie

Ingredients	Quantity	Method
Greek yogurt - low fat, low sugar	170g or 6oz	Put all in a jug or nutri-bullet and biltz. Pour into a glass and drink!
Banana - Ripe	1 medium	
Peanut Butter - smooth	2 Tb	

For those without diabetes, you can add a teaspoon of honey for taste.

Nutritional Analysis Per Serving

USA: Energy (kj/kcal): 1669 (399) Protein (g): 25, Carbohydrate (g): 31, Sugar (g): 24, Total Fat (g): 5.3, Sodium (mg): 64, Dietary Fiber (g): 4.6

Australia: Energy (kj/kcal): 1907 (456) Protein (g): 23, Carbohydrate (g): 38, Sugar (g): 30, Total Fat (g): 20, Sodium (mg): 218, Dietary Fiber (g): 8

New Zealand: Energy (kj/kcal): 2119 (506), Protein (g): 28, Carbohydrate (g): 33, Sugar (g): 25, Total Fat (g): 29, Sodium (mg): 86, Dietary Fiber (g): 7.9

Peachy Smoothie

Ingredients	Quantity	Method
Greek yogurt - low fat, low sugar	170g or 6oz	Put all in a jug or nutri-bullet and biltz. Pour into a glass and drink!
Peaches, canned, drained	1 Cup	
Skim milk powder	1 Tb	

For those without diabetes, you can add a teaspoon of honey for taste.

Nutritional Analysis Per Serving

USA: Energy (kj/kcal): 1283 (307); Protein (g): 23, Carbohydrate (g): 30, Sugar (g): 30, Total Fat (g): 4, Sodium (mg): 64, Dietary Fiber (g): 3.7

Australia: Energy (kj/kcal): 1613 (386) Protein (g): 25, Carbohydrate (g): 48, Sugar (g): 48, Total Fat (g): 5.8, Sodium (mg):347, Dietary Fiber (g): 10.2

New Zealand: Energy (kj/kcal): 1631 (317), Protein (g): 29, Carbohydrate (g): 39, Sugar (g): 39, Total Fat (g): 7.5, Sodium (mg): 165, Dietary Fiber (g): 3.2

Soup Recipes

These recipes are for 4 servings. You can always cool down extra soup and freeze it for later consumption. Remember to label your container with what it is and the date.

Crème of Chicken Soup

Ingredients	Quantity	Ingredients	Quantity
Garlic Infused Oil	1 Tb	Potatoes - peeled, diced	1 medium
Onion Infused Oil	1 Tb	Plain Flour	2 Tb
Diced Chicken Pieces (or tenderloin)	340g or ¾ pound	Chicken Broth	1 cup
Milk	2 cups	Cream (heavy) or Coconut Cream	½ cup
Parsley	1 large bunch	Water	1 cup
Carrot	2 large - diced	Salt & Pepper to taste	

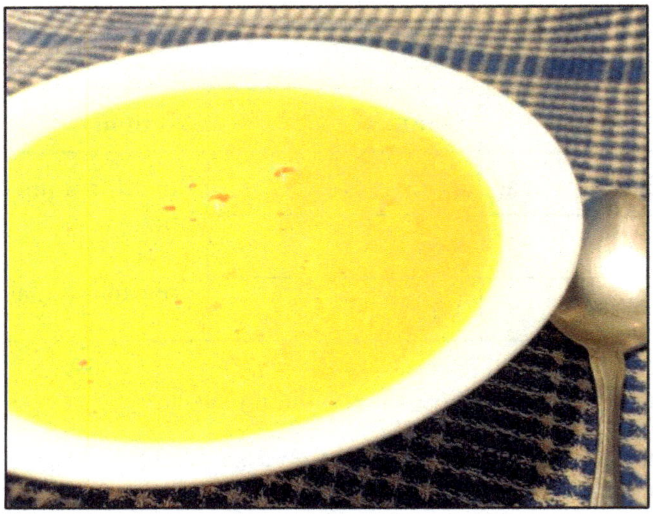

1. To make your own broth, in a pot, add four chicken frames to 3 cups of water, allow to boil and then turn own to slowly simmer for an hour to 90 minutes. Take off the stove.
2. Allow to cool down.
3. Pour out the broth into clean jug. Discard frame (unless there is meat on the frames, you can remove the meat to add to the soup).

A good quality broth made from chicken bones will have collagen in the water and that is great for gut healing.

Make Parsley Water

This is to give more flavor and note that parsley is full of goodness that is great for health and immunity.
1. Chop parsley including stalk and put into a pot of water (1 cup). I also added in 1 Tablespoon of Thyme and 1 Tablespoon to Rosemary (for flavor).
2. Simmer for 15 minutes.

3. Remove from the stove.
4. Use a handheld stick blender if you have one or put into a blender and blend to make a pureed liquid.
5. Once done, use a sieve and just get the green parsley juice.

Cooking Creme of Chicken
1. In a pot, heat the garlic infused oil and the onion infused oil, Add diced chicken pieces and lightly cook.
2. Add chicken broth, parsley water, diced carrots & diced pumpkin.
3. Cook in low heat for an hour, stirring occasionally.
4. Add salt & pepper to taste.
5. Check to see that the potato is cooked.
6. Remove pot from heat.
7. Use a stick blender to puree the soup to make creme of chicken soup.
8. Put back on stove to simmer.
9. Add cream, stir cream in and simmer for a few minutes.

Extra Ideas

I played with this above recipe to show how you can increase your options using the above recipe as a base idea.

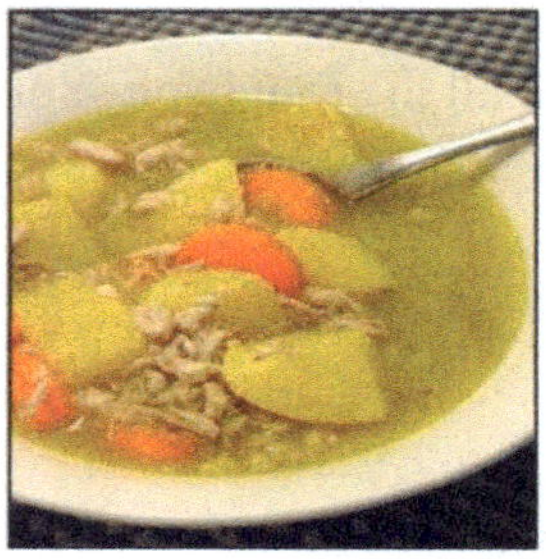	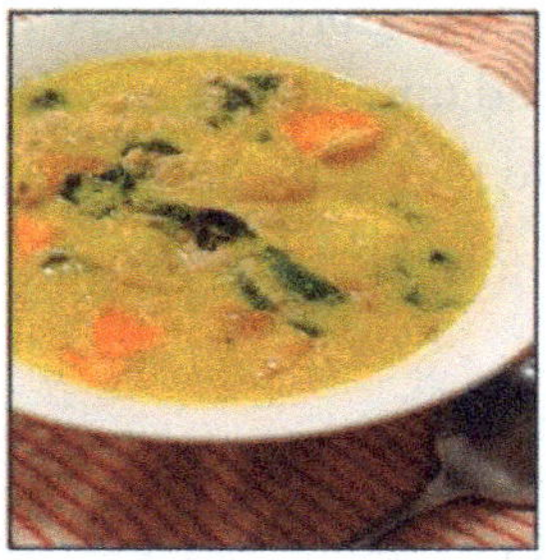	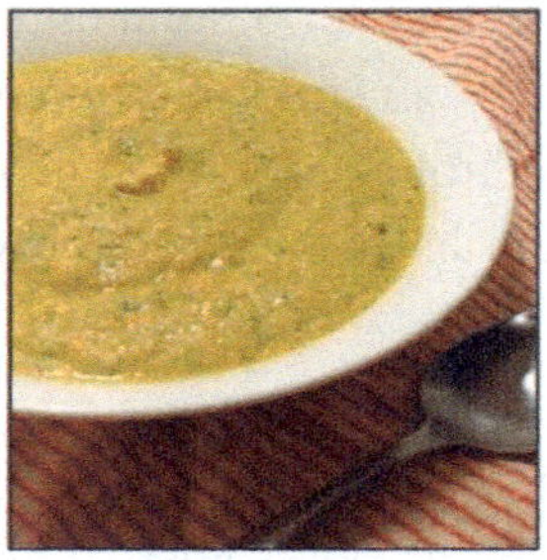
I did not puree the soup, left it with its component whole. My 11 year old liked this one the best as she said it had layers of flavour compared to the others.	In this one, I added sliced spinach (taking the stalks off first to decrease roughage). Tasted great to me but spinach had a slimy feel to it.	Pureed soup that had spinach in it. It tasted great and looked awesome too. But my 11 year old did not like it!

Nutritional Analysis Per Serving

USA: Energy (kj/kcal): 1696 (405) Protein (g): 25, Carbohydrate (g): 20, Sugar (g): 11.5, Total Fat (g): 25 Sodium (mg): 472, Dietary Fiber (g): 1.3

Australia: Energy (kj/kcal): 1771 (423) Protein (g): 22, Carbohydrate (g): 13, Sugar (g): 13, Total Fat (g): 27, Sodium (mg): 403, Dietary Fiber (g): 1.3

New Zealand: Energy (kj/kcal): 1680 (404), Protein (g): 24, Carbohydrate (g): 17.5, Sugar (g): 11 Total Fat (g): 26, Sodium (mg): 496, Dietary Fiber (g): 0.9

Crème of Pumpkin Soup

Ingredient	Quantity	Ingredient	Quantity
Pumpkin – deseeded	1kg or 2.2 lb	Nutmeg - ground	2 tsp
Garlic Crush	1 Tb (8cloves)	Cumin	2 tsp
Onion – diced	1 large	Salt & Pepper to taste	
Oil	3 Tb	Cream	½ cup
Chicken/Vegetable Stock or Broth	3 cups	Salt & Pepper to taste	
Water	1 cup		

Method

Prepare the base liquid.

1. In a large pot, heat oil.
2. Add onion and fry till onion is clear.
3. Add crushed garlic.
4. Simmer to cook until garlic is cooked.
5. Add vegetable/chicken stock and water to this.
6. Allow to simmer for 5 minutes.
7. Take pot off stove and run the liquid through a hand-held stick blender to finely puree all the onion/garlic mix through the mixture.
8. Put back on stove for 5 minutes and bring mixture to almost boiling temperature.
9. Remove pot from stove and run the liquid through a sieve to remove all the roughage. You can press out the liquid through the sieve and discard the left-over roughage.
10. Put liquid back in the pot and back on the stove.

Add in pumpkin

1. Cut pumpkin into large slice, remove skin and cut into 3 -3.5cm cubes.
2. Add pumpkin and simmer for 55 minutes until pumpkin is tender.
3. Remove from heat and use blender to puree the soup.
4. Add in cup of cream, salt, and pepper.

Ladle to serve.

Nutritional Analysis Per Serving

USA: Energy (kj/kcal): 1456 (348) Protein (g): 8, Carbohydrate (g): 10.9 Sugar (g): 1, Total Fat (g): 281, Sodium (mg): 281, Dietary Fiber (g): 1.3

Australia: Energy (kj/kcal): 1116 (267) Protein (g): 6.4, Carbohydrate (g): 19, Sugar (g): 14, Total Fat (g): 17, Sodium (mg): 689, Dietary Fiber (g): 1.1

New Zealand: Energy (kj/kcal): 1021 (244), Protein (g): 3.4, Carbohydrate (g): 19, Sugar (g): 13, Total Fat (g): 17, Sodium (mg): 1060, Dietary Fiber (g): 3.4

Crème of Tomato Soup

Ingredient	Quantity	Ingredient	Quantity
Canned Diced Tomato	1 can	Onion Infused Oil	1 Tb
Chicken or Vegetable Broth	1 cup	Cream	½ cup
Water	1 cup	Corn flour / Flour	1 Tb
Italian Herb Infused Oil	1 Tb	Sugar (optional)	1 Tb
Garlic Infused Oil	1 Tb	Salt & Pepper to taste	

Method

1. In a pot, add chicken or vegetable stock. Add in corn flour/flour for thickening. Whisk this in.
2. Add the oils and diced canned tomato to the pot. Add sugar (if need for a sweeter flavor but not for those with diabetes).
3. Allow to boil and then simmer for 10 minutes.
4. Take off stove.
5. Use a blender to puree.
6. Pass through sieve into a jug.
7. Add in cream.

Nutritional Analysis Per Serving

USA: Energy (kj/kcal): 1696 (405), Protein (g): 25, Carbohydrate (g): 20, Sugar (g): 12, Total Fat (g): 25, Sodium (mg): 472, Dietary Fiber (g): 1.3

Australia: Energy (kj/kcal): 1771 (423) Protein (g): 24.4, Carbohydrate (g): 22, Sugar (g): 13, Total Fat (g): 27, Sodium (mg): 401, Dietary Fiber (g): 1.1

New Zealand: Energy (kj/kcal): 1680 (401), Protein (g): 24, Carbohydrate (g): 18, Sugar (g): 11, Total Fat (g): 26, Sodium (mg): 496, Dietary Fiber (g): 0.9

Adaptations For Vegan Diet

A vegan diet needs to meet its protein through use of nuts, seeds, lentils, legumes, beans, chickpeas, tempeh, tofu etc.

Since a low roughage diet means removing any harsh unbroken fibers, the following adaptations need to be made to meet the daily protein requirement:

1. Use smooth nut butter instead of nuts.

2. For lentils and legumes:

- use those that have no skin, such as red and yellow lentils.
- soak these overnight to allow the fibers to become softer with water. Remove water in the morning.
- smooth blend soups to ensure that every component is broken down.
- note that lentils, legumes etc. can cause bloating. Thus monitor the symptoms of bloating. It may be that your gut is unable to digest these at present.

3. Use tempeh and tofu as protein options. You could try marinating these overnight.

4. Chewing food till smooth in your mouth before swallowing is recommended.

5. Use protein powers like pea protein isolate where possible. Aim for 20g to 30g of protein for each meal.

Tofu (100g) has around 12g of protein.

Tempeh (100g) has 18g of protein.

Peanut butter (1Tb) has 3g of protein.

You can adapt some of the recipes given by substituting with a suitable plant protein option.

Dinner Recipes

Week 1: Day 1: Citrus Salmon with Pea Puree with Mashed Sweet Potato

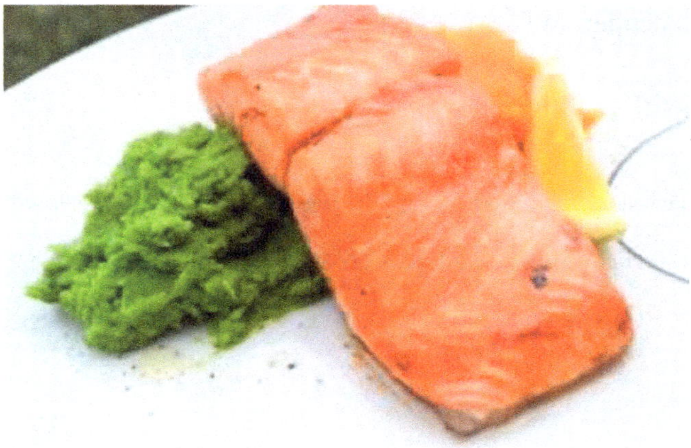

Ingredient	Quantity	Ingredient	Quantity
Garlic Infused Oil	1 Tb	Orange Juice	2 Tb
Onion Infused Oil	1 Tb	Salt, Table	1 dash
Salmon Steak	2 fillets (1 fillet: 100g/3.5 oz)	Peas	1 cup
		Sweet Potato, Peeled, Diced	1 medium size
		Milk, Standard	2 Tb
Lemon Juice	1 lemon yield	Margarine	1 heaped Tb
Honey	1 Tb	Salt & Pepper To Taste	

Method

1. In a bowl, mix garlic infused oil, onion infused oil, lemon juice, salt, and honey.
2. Heat a non-stick frying pan on medium heat.
3. Spray on oil.
4. Grill salmon with skin down for 10 – 15 minutes, basting with the marinade made above every 3 minutes. Turn over the last minute and grill off (however, you may not want to do that). Ensure that the salmon flakes with a fork.
5. Take of heat.
6. Serve with pureed peas and mashed potato.

To prepare pureed peas:

1. Defrost frozen peas.
2. Cook in boiling hot water till very soft.
3. Remove pan from heat. Drain water off. Using a blender, blend till pureed.
4. Using a sieve, strain fibrous component from soft puree. Discard fibrous residue.
5. Serve soft puree with meal.

To prepare mashed kumara or sweet potato

1. In a pot with water, add diced sweet potato and bring water to boil.

2. Turn down heat and simmer till sweet potato is cooked.
3. When cooked, turn element off.
4. Drain water from sweet potato.
5. Add margarine, salt and pepper, milk.
6. Mash until smooth.

Serve for dinner. Bon appétit!

Nutritional Analysis Per Serving

USA: Energy (kj/kcal): 2708 (647) Protein (g): 28, Carbohydrate (g): 40, Sugar (g): 26, Total Fat (g): 40, Sodium (mg): 1023, Dietary Fiber (g): 5.5

Australia: Energy (kj/kcal): 1970 (471) Protein (g): 25, Carbohydrate (g): 32, Sugar (g): 15, Total Fat (g): 32, Sodium (mg): 131, Dietary Fiber (g): 4.3

New Zealand: Energy (kj/kcal): 2362 (595), Protein (g): 24, Carbohydrate (g): 28, Sugar (g): 14, Total Fat (g): 10, Sodium (mg): 160, Dietary Fiber (g): 3.0

Week 1: Day 2: Beef Burger

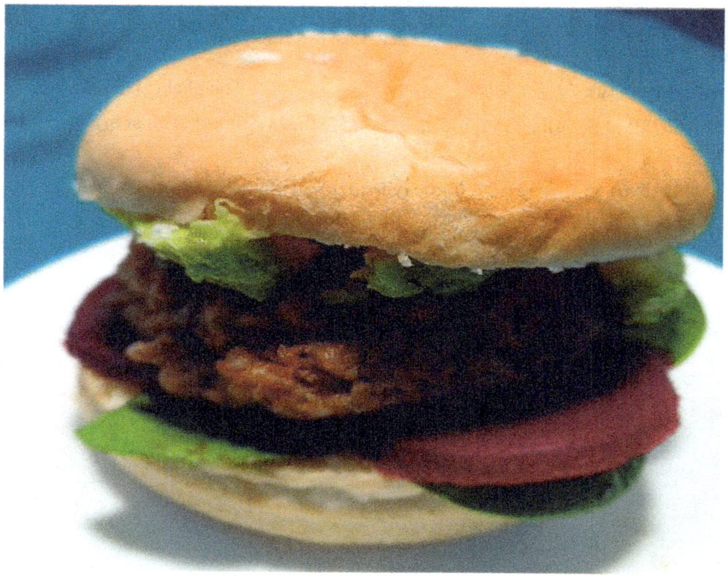

Ingredient	Quantity	Ingredient	Quantity
Olive Oil	2 Tb	Beetroot - canned, drained, dried	8 slices
Beef Mince	200g (7oz)	Baby Spinach	½ cup
Paprika	¼ tsp	Egg	1
Ground Cumin	¼ tsp	Flour	6 Tb
Avocado	½	Salt to taste	
Mayonnaise	2 Tb	Burger Buns	2

Method

To make mince patties.
1. In a bowl, add mince, egg, paprika, salt, cumin powder, and flour together and mix well.
2. Divide the mixture for two patties. Pat and shape in patty shapes.
3. Heat oil in a skillet / pan. Place patties on the pan and cook for 5 minutes on each side on low heat, checking to see that it is cooked. When cooked, put aside on a plate.

Prepare the salad component
1. Take of stalks of baby spinach.
2. Slice avocado into 8 slices
3. Use a paper towel to dry out the beetroot.

Prepare Beef Burger
1. Cut burger into half.
2. Lightly grill the exposed side of the burger for slight crunch.
3. Remove from being under a grill.
4. Place each burger on a plate to assemble.
5. On the bottom piece, spread mayonnaise, then layer spinach leaves, beetroot, beef patty, sliced avocado (4 per burger).

6. Cover with burger bun top half and eat! Dig in!

Nutritional Analysis Per Serving

USA: Energy (kj/kcal): 2768 (662) Protein (g): 22, Carbohydrate (g): 17, Sugar (g): 7, Total Fat (g): 56, Sodium (mg): 468.9, Dietary Fiber (g): 7

Australia: Energy (kj/kcal): 2790 (667) Protein (g): 29, Carbohydrate (g): 52, Sugar (g): 7, Total Fat (g): 56, Sodium (mg): 469, Dietary Fiber (g): 6.8

New Zealand: Energy (kj/kcal): 2495 (596), Protein (g): 27, Carbohydrate (g): 51, Sugar (g): 11, Total Fat (g): 34, Sodium (mg): 657, Dietary Fiber (g): 7.4

Week 1: Day 3: Apricot Chicken

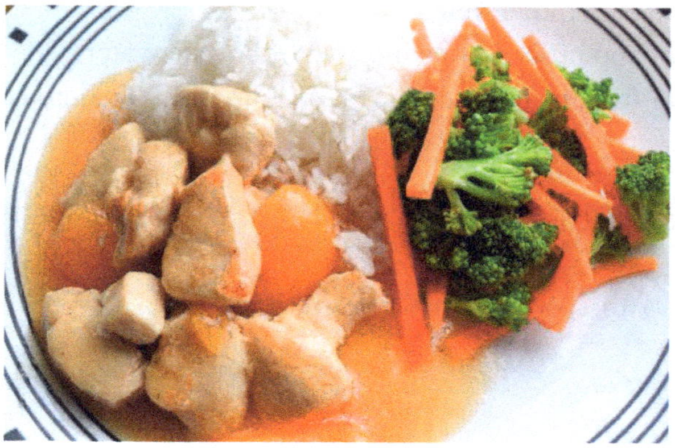

Ingredient	Quantity	Ingredient	Quantity
Diced Boneless Chicken	200g / 7oz	Tomato Sauce	1 Tb
Apricots, Canned, With Juice- Quartered	100g / 3.5 oz	Garlic Oil	2 Tb
		Rice	1 cup
Water	¼ cup	Broccoli	4 florets
Corn flour	2 Tb	Carrot, Peeled, Diced	1 large
Infused Onion Oil	2 Tb		
Salt Table	1 dash		

Method

To cook apricot chicken

1. Heat garlic oil and infused onion oil in a non-stick pan.
2. Add diced chicken and seal sides.
3. Add water, salt, tomato sauce and simmer for 10-15 minutes until the chicken is almost cooked.
4. Add apricots
5. Simmer for another 10 minutes.
6. If the liquid is too thin, add corn flour in a little bit of water and make a roux. Add to the chicken mix to thicken.
7. Simmer low for another 5 minutes. Turn off heat.

To cook rice in the microwave

1. Put rice in microwaveable dish
2. Wash 3 times.
3. Add water to rice. The measurement of water is done like this. Put your pointer finger to the top of the rice. Add water to the first knuckle.
4. Microwave on high for 9 minutes.
5. Take out and let it sit for 3 minutes.
6. Check that rice is cooked by pressing a flake in-between your finger and your thumb.
7. If still uncooked, add a bit more water and cook for further 2-3 minutes.

To prepare vegetables

1. Regarding broccoli – use tips, remove stems.
2. Steam or cook diced carrot and broccoli tips in a pan of boiling water.
3. When cooked, remove pan from heat, drain and serve with meal. Delicious!

Nutritional Analysis Per Serving

USA: Energy (kj/kcal): 1964 (469), Protein (g): 25, Carbohydrate (g): 39, Sugar (g): 2, Total Fat (g): 16, Sodium (mg): 361, Dietary Fiber (g): 3

Australia: Energy (kj/kcal): 2650 (633) Protein (g): 29, Carbohydrate (g): 66, Sugar (g): 9, Total Fat (g):27, Sodium (mg): 546, Dietary Fiber (g): 7.3

New Zealand: Energy (kj/kcal): 3309 (794), Protein (g): 31, Carbohydrate (g): 106, Sugar (g): 12, Total Fat (g): 27, Sodium (mg): 546, Dietary Fiber (g): 4.7

Week 1: Day 4: Creamy Prawn Pasta

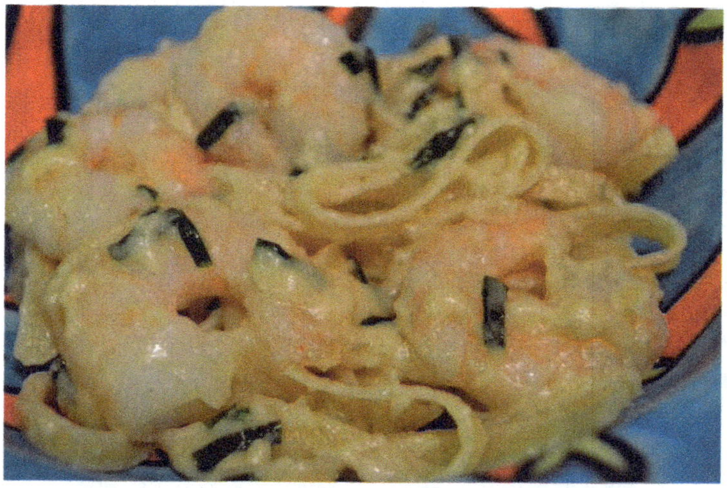

Ingredient	Quantity	Ingredient	Quantity
Prawn, Shelled	280g / 10oz	Whole Milk	½ cup
Garlic Oil	1 Tb	Ground Black Pepper	1 dash
Infused Onion Oil	1 Tb	Linguine pasta	170g / 6 oz
Corn flour	2 tsp	Lemon Juice	1 lemon yields

Method

1. Clean prawn to just flesh.
2. Cook linguini in a large saucepan of boiling, salted water according to packet directions. Add 3. peas 2 minutes before end of cooking time.
4. Drain and return to pan to keep warm.
5. Meanwhile, heat oil in a frying pan on high. Cook prawns, stirring for 2 minutes, until pink.
6. Stir in garlic, lemon juice. remove from heat.
7. In a separate pan, heat oil, make a roux using corn flour and milk.
8. Add prawn to this. Mix.
9. Pour over linguini. Mix.

Have a great meal!

Nutritional Analysis Per Serving

USA: Energy (kj/kcal): 1128 (270), Protein (g): 21, Carbohydrate (g): 5, Sugar (g): 4, Total Fat (g): 13, Sodium (mg): 841, Dietary Fiber (g): 0.5

Australia: Energy (kj/kcal): 2189 (523) Protein (g): 35, Carbohydrate (g): 65, Sugar (g): 2, Total Fat (g):40, Sodium (mg): 509, Dietary Fiber (g): 3

New Zealand: Energy (kj/kcal): 1128 (370), Protein (g): 21, Carbohydrate (g): 5, Sugar (g): 4, Total Fat (g): 13, Sodium (mg): 841, Dietary Fiber (g): 0.5

Week 1: Day 5: Braised Lamb Chop with Rice

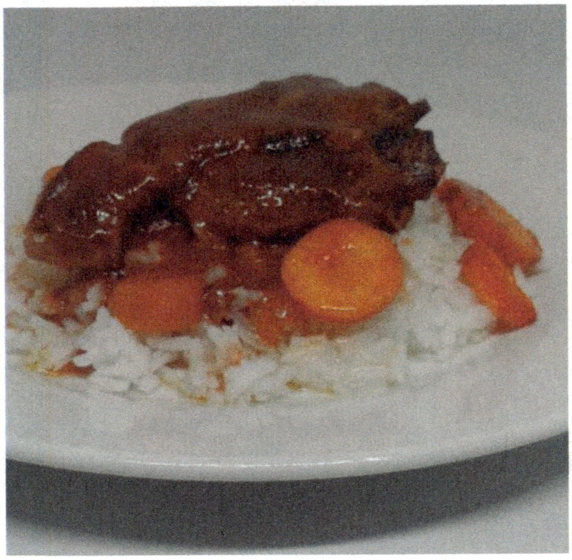

Ingredient	Quantity	Ingredient	Quantity
Rice	½ cup	Lamb Loin Chops	230g / ½ pound
Garlic Oil	1 Tb	Tomato Paste	2 Tb
Rosemary Leaves, Dried	1 tsp.	Water	4 Tb
Water	2 Tb	Lemon Juice	1 lemon yields
Carrot	1 large		

Method

Preheat oven at 150ºC/300ºF

Cook rice in the microwave

1. Put rice in microwaveable dish,
2. Wash 3 times.
3. Add 1 cup water to rice.
4. Microwave on high for 10 minutes.
5. Take out and let it sit for 3 minutes.
6. Check that the rice is cooked by pressing a flake in-between your finger and your thumb.
7. If still uncooked, add a bit more water and cook for further 2-3 minutes.

Cook braised lamb chop

1. Pound rosemary to remove juice from leaves.
2. Once the juice has separated from leave, add 2 tsp of water and mix.
3. Pour mixture through a sieve to remove all debris and roughage.
4. In a cup, mix tomato paste, rosemary juice, water, and corn flour.
5. In a casserole dish, pour garlic infused oil and onion infused oil.
6. Lay lamb chops in the casserole dish. Lay carrot on top. And pour the tomato mix on top.
7. Bake for 45 minutes. Check to see that the meat is cooked.
8. Serve with steamed rice.

Relish every bite!

<u>Nutritional Analysis Per Serving</u>
USA: Energy (kj/kcal): 1895 (453), Protein (g): 27, Carbohydrate (g): 39, Sugar (g):5, Total Fat (g): 19, Sodium (mg): 312, Dietary Fiber (g): 4
Australia: Energy (kj/kcal): 2485 (28) Protein (g): 28, Carbohydrate (g): 28, Sugar (g): 9, Total Fat (g):33, Sodium (mg): 116, Dietary Fiber (g): 4
New Zealand: Energy (kj/kcal): 3811 (911), Protein (g): 30, Carbohydrate (g): 36, Sugar (g): 5, Total Fat (g): 19, Sodium (mg): 99, Dietary Fiber (g): 3

Week 1: Day 6: Beef Meatball in Tortilla Wrap with Cucumber, Carrot

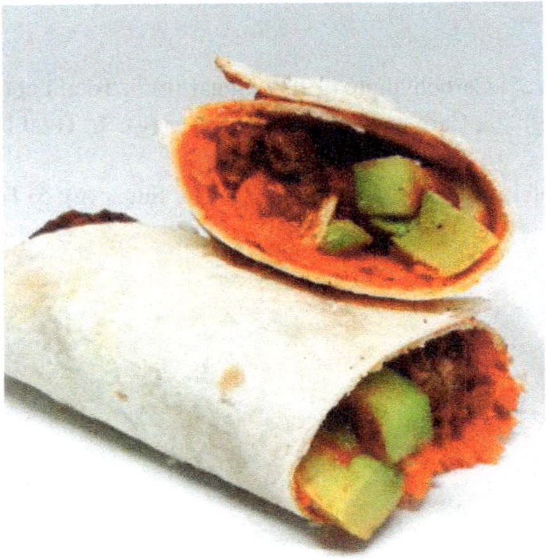

Ingredient	Quantity	Ingredient	Quantity
Olive Oil	4 Tb	Worcestershire Sauce	1 tsp
Beef Mince – Lean	200g / 7 oz	Salt	To taste
Bread Crumbs – Dry	3 Tb	Ready Made Bolognaise Sauce	½ can (100g / 3.5 oz)
Garam Masala	¾ tsp	Tortilla Wrap – Ready Made	2
Nutmeg- Ground	½ tsp	Cucumber (Deseeded, Peeled)	½ medium cucumber
White Pepper	½ tsp	Carrot	1 medium size
Onion Infused Oil	1 tsp	Avocado	½ medium size
Garlic Infused Oil	1 tsp		

Method

To make meatballs

1. Mix all ingredients (except the sunflower oil) together.
2. Roll into 20g balls – makes 12 balls.
3. Place on a tray.
4. Heat sunflower oil in frying pan.
5. Gently put each meatball in the frying pan and cook under low heat, turning regularly to ensure even cooking.
6. When cooked, remove, and put on clean plate.

Bolognaise sauce: need a sieve.

I used readymade bottled bolognaise sauce.

1. Pour bolognaise sauce through a sieve to remove all big particles, to collect a smooth sauce in a bottom container.
2. Discard all the sieved particles.
3. In a pot, heat the sieved bolognaise sauce.
4. Add the cooked lamb meatballs to the sauce and simmer for 5 minutes in low heat.

Prepare the tortilla meal

1. Place a tortilla wrap on plate.
2. Layer across grated carrot, sliced cucumber, take 5 meatballs and put side by side length wise on the vegetable layer.
3. Add sliced avocado on top.
4. Roll the side of the wrap together to encase.
5. Cut across in half in the center.

Wishing you a tasty meal!

Nutritional Analysis Per Serving

USA: Energy (kj/kcal): 2328 (556), Protein (g): 29, Carbohydrate (g): 29, Sugar (g): 4, Total Fat (g): 28, Sodium (mg): 1147, Dietary Fiber (g): 8

Australia: Energy (kj/kcal): 2167 (518) Protein (g): 30, Carbohydrate (g): 47, Sugar (g):10, Total Fat (g):22, Sodium (mg): 572 Dietary Fiber (g): 7

New Zealand: Energy (kj/kcal): 2078 (497), Protein (g): 27, Carbohydrate (g): 30, Sugar (g): 5, Total Fat (g): 30, Sodium (mg): 168, Dietary Fiber (g): 7.5

Week 1: Day 7: Roast Pork, Mashed Potato, Boiled Pumpkin, Silverbeet / Swiss Chard

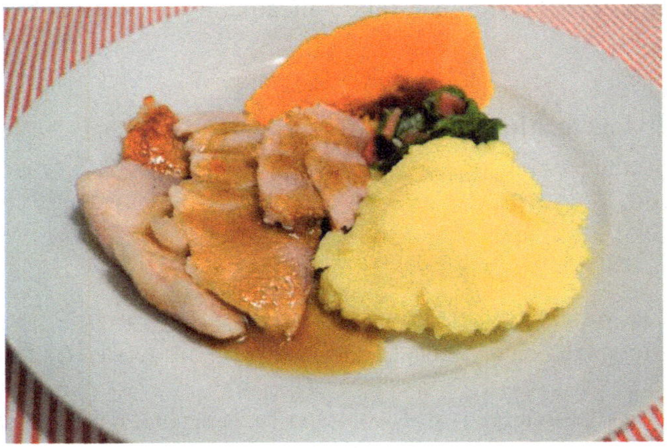

Ingredient	Quantity	Ingredient	Quantity
Olive Oil	1Tb	Pumpkin	100g / 3.5 oz
Pork Shoulder Roast	200g	Silverbeet	100g / 3.5 oz
Salt	Pinch	Milk	2 Tb
Potato, Diced	1 medium	Margarine /Butter	1 Tb
Salt & Pepper to Taste.			

Method

Pre-heat oven to 205°C/400°F

1. Place pork shoulder roast on rack in a roasting dish. Rub salt on the skin.
2. Roast for 15 minutes. Reduce temperature to 150°C/300°F and roast further for 45 minutes.
3. Pork is cooked when internal temperature reaches at least 71°C/160°F
4. Remove from oven and set aside to rest.
5. Boil diced potatoes.
6. In separate pots, boil pumpkin and silver beet. When cooked, drain off water.
7. Drain and mash with milk and margarine.
8. Season with salt and pepper.

Here's to good food and good company!

Nutritional Analysis Per Serving

USA: Energy (kj/kcal): 1353 (323), Protein (g): 17, Carbohydrate (g): 18, Sugar (g): 0.3, Total Fat (g): 24, Sodium (mg): 1681, Dietary Fiber (g): 3

Australia: Energy (kj/kcal): 1001 (239) Protein (g): 23, Carbohydrate (g): 16, Sugar (g): 3, Total Fat (g):9, Sodium (mg): 404, Dietary Fiber (g): 3

New Zealand: Energy (kj/kcal): 1001 (239), Protein (g): 23, Carbohydrate (g): 16, Sugar (g): 6, Total Fat (g): 9, Sodium (mg): 404, Dietary Fiber (g): 3

Week 2: Day 1: Scotch Fillet, Mashed Potato with Steamed Pumpkin & Broccoli

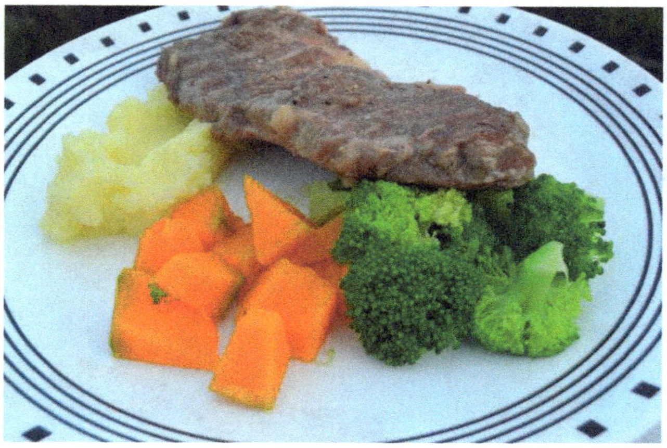

Ingredient	Quantity	Ingredient	Quantity
Scotch Fillet	240g	Margarine / Butter	1 Tb
Olive Oil	1 tsp	Salt	To taste
Salt	Dash	Pumpkin	100g
Potato, Peeled	160g	Broccoli	6 florets
Milk	1 Tb		

Method

Cook scotch fillet

1. Heat oil in non-stick pan on high heat.
2. Rub salt on the scotch fillet and cook as follows: cook 2 minutes each side for rare, 3-4 mins each side for medium-rare and 4-6 mins each side for medium. For well done, cook for 2-4 minutes each side, then turn the heat down and cook for another 4-6 minutes.
3. When cooked, remove, cover with foil and rest for a few minutes (5-7 minutes), remove foil, cut and serve.

To prepare the vegetables

1. Boil diced potato in water until soft. Drain water off when cooked.
2. Mash potato with milk, margarine/butter and salt until smooth.
3. Similarly boil peeled diced pumpkin until soft, drain water off when cooked.
4. Steam or boil broccoli tips. Drain water.
5. Plate up.

Hope it hits the spot!

Nutritional Analysis Per Serving

USA: Energy (kj/kcal): 1549 (370), Protein (g): 36, Carbohydrate (g): 18, Sugar (g): 1, Total Fat (g): 16, Sodium (mg): 343, Dietary Fiber (g): 4

Australia: Energy (kj/kcal): 1351 (323) Protein (g): 38, Carbohydrate (g): 14, Sugar (g): 4, Total Fat (g):12, Sodium (mg): 347, Dietary Fiber (g): 3

New Zealand: Energy (kj/kcal): 1549 (370), Protein (g): 36, Carbohydrate (g): 18, Sugar (g): 1, Total Fat (g): 5, Sodium (mg): 343, Dietary Fiber (g): 4

Week 2: Day 2: Bacon Egg Potato Top Pie

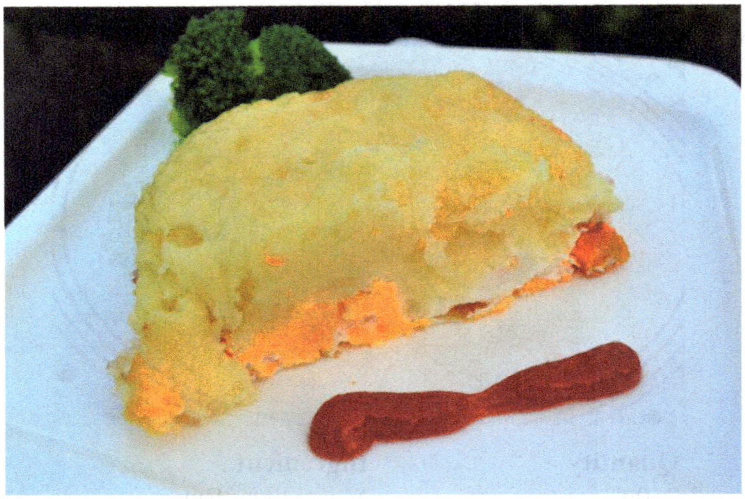

Ingredient	Quantity	Ingredient	Quantity
Diced Shoulder Bacon Pieces (Remove Rind)	200g / 7 oz	Whole Milk	3 Tb
Whole Egg	4 small eggs	Ground Black Pepper	1 dash
Ground White Pepper	¼ tsp	Grated Cheese	60g or 2 oz
Steamed Diced Carrot	1/2 cup	Tomato Sauce	4 Tb
Peeled Diced Medium Potato	170g / 6 oz	Broccoli tip	1 large floret

Method

1. Boil and mash diced potato. Add milk, seasonings to taste.

Turn oven to 180°C/350°F

1. In a small flan dish, place steamed diced carrot
2. Break whole egg on the mixed vegetable.
3. Add ground white pepper to taste
4. Layer mashed potato on top.
5. Sprinkle cheese on top
6. Place in oven and cook for 20 minutes, checking in the end with a knife prick to see that the egg is cooked. If it is not, cook for another 5-10 minutes.
7. Remove from the oven when cooked, slice and serve hot.

Take your time and enjoy!

Nutritional Analysis Per Serving

USA: Energy (kj/kcal): 2975 (711), Protein (g): 30, Carbohydrate (g): 23, Sugar (g): 6, Total Fat (g): 52, Sodium (mg): 1279, Dietary Fiber (g): 4

Australia: Energy (kj/kcal): 1776 (424) Protein (g): 28, Carbohydrate (g): 20, Sugar (g): 2, Total Fat (g):24, Sodium (mg): 1053, Dietary Fiber (g): 10

New Zealand: Energy (kj/kcal): 4076 (974), Protein (g): 26, Carbohydrate (g): 16, Sugar (g): 2, Total Fat (g): 38.3, Sod um (mg): 828, Dietary Fiber (g): 2

Week 2: Day 3: Moroccan Lamb Shank with Sweet Potato or Kumara, Swiss Chard/Silverbeet, Pumpkin

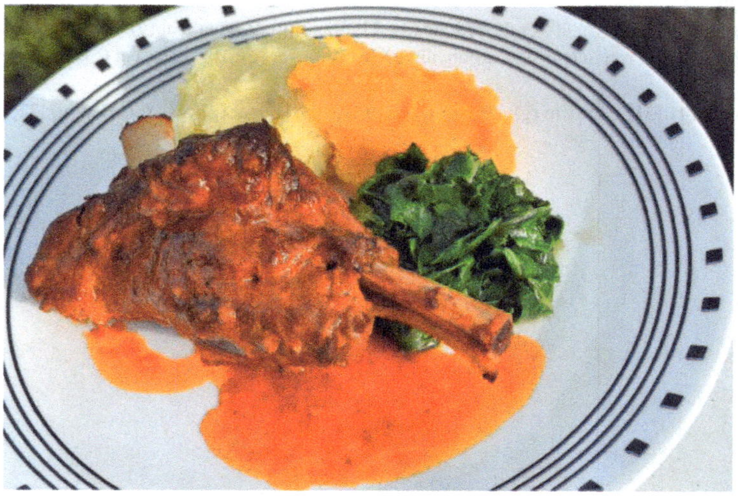

Ingredient	Quantity	Ingredient	Quantity
Garlic Oil	1 Tb	Salt	Dash
Infused Onion Oil	1 Tb	Water	1 cup
Lamb Shank	2 shanks	Potato, Medium, Peeled	200g / 7 oz
Ground Cumin Seed	½ tsp	Milk, Standard	4 Tb
Coriander Powder	½ tsp	Swiss Chard / Silverbeet	140g / 5 oz
Turmeric	1 tsp	Pumpkin (Skinless, Seedless, Diced)	120g / 4 oz
Tomato paste	3 Tb		

Method

To prepare mashed potato

1. Boil diced potato till soft.
2. Drain off water.
3. Mash with milk and add seasoning

To cook Moroccan Lamb Shank

1. Heat infused oil in a frying pan.
2. Seal the lamb shank to intensify taste. Remove from heat.
3. In a bowl, mix tomato paste, tomato paste, coriander powder, turmeric, and water.
4. Turn on a slow cooker to high. Add lamb shank, pour tomato mix on this. Add salt to taste
5. Slow cook for 4-6 hours, turning the lamb shank couple of times during this period.

To prepare vegetables

1. Take required amount of Silverbeet/Swiss chard. Remove soft leafy part from white stalk.
2. Add to a pot of boiling water. Simmer till soft. Drain and serve with meal.
3. Boil pumpkin till soft. Drain and serve with meal. When cooked, serve with rice.

Hope it’s as delicious as it looks!

<u>Nutritional Analysis Per Serving</u>

USA: Energy (kj/kcal): 2690 (643), Protein (g): 49, Carbohydrate (g): 27, Sugar (g): 9, Total Fat (g): 26, Sodium (mg): 1182, Dietary Fiber (g): 7
Australia: Energy (kj/kcal): 2280 (545) Protein (g): 39, Carbohydrate (g): 34, Sugar (g): 10, Total Fat (g):8, Sodium (mg): 671, Dietary Fiber (g): 8
New Zealand: Energy (kj/kcal): 2141 (512), Protein (g): 49, Carbohydrate (g): 28, Sugar (g): 13, Total Fat (g): 22, Sodium (mg): 1182, Dietary Fiber (g): 5

Week 2: Day 4: Pan Fried Fish with Lemon Slice, Mashed Potato, Broccoli

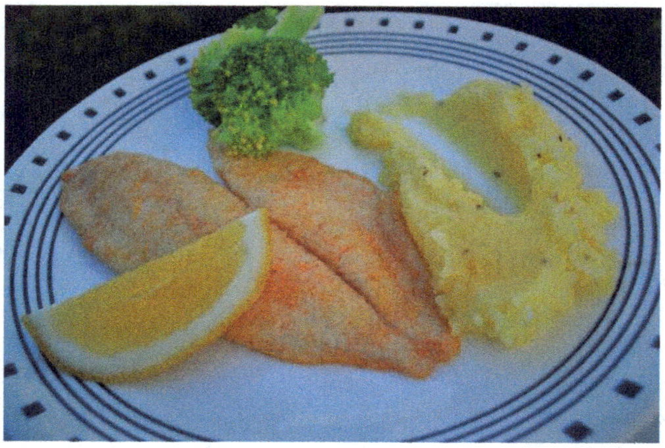

Ingredient	Quantity	Ingredient	Quantity
Fish Fillet	2 fillets (1 fillet: 120g or 4 oz)	Salt, Table	½ tsp
Olive Oil	1 Tb	Lemon Slice	4 wedges
Flour	4 Tb	Potato, Peeled	1 medium (200g/ 7oz)
Ground Cumin	¼ tsp	Milk, Standard	2 Tb
Paprika Powder	¼ tsp	Salt	Dash
Ground Coriander	¼ tsp	Ground Pepper	Dash
		Broccoli Tip	140g

Method

To cook fish fillet

1. Mix flour, paprika, cumin, coriander together.
2. Coat fish fillet with the flour mixture.
3. Heat oil in shallow fry pan. Pan fry for few minutes on each side, to cook and seal the fish. Should have a reddish golden coating.
4. Remove from pan and servings of with lemon wedges with vegetables

To prepare the vegetables

1. Boil peeled diced potato till soft. Drain off water, add salt, milk and ground pepper and mash till smooth.
2. Boil broccoli tip. When cooked, drain off water.

Treat yourself to this!

Nutritional Analysis Per Serving

USA: Energy (kj/kcal): 1159 (227), Protein (g): 23, Carbohydrate (g): 18, Sugar (g): 1, Total Fat (g): 10, Sodium (mg): 435, Dietary Fiber (g): 5

Australia: Energy (kj/kcal): 1534 (367) Protein (g): 27, Carbohydrate (g): 40, Sugar (g): 3, Total Fat (g): 12, Sodium (mg): 627, Dietary Fiber (g): 5

New Zealand: Energy (kj/kcal): 2153 (514), Protein (g): 32, Carbohydrate (g): 40, Sugar (g): 3, Total Fat (g): 6, Sodium (mg): 578 , Dietary Fiber (g): 4

Week 2: Day 5: Chicken in Basil Sauce

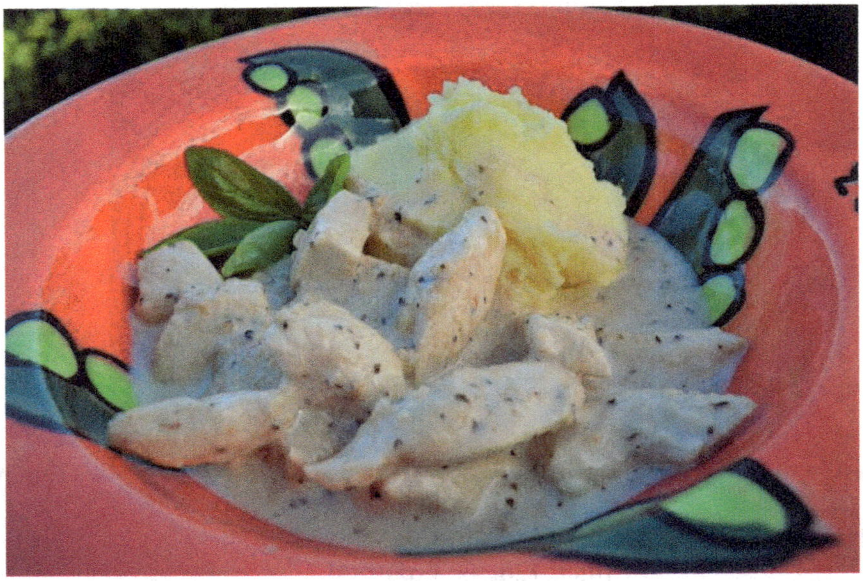

Ingredients	Quantity	Ingredients	Quantity
Margarine	1 Tb	Diced Chicken	220g/8oz
Corn Flour	2 tsp	Infused Garlic Oil	1 tsp
Milk	100 mL	Infused Onion Oil	2 tsp
Ground Dried Basil	1 Tb	Potato, Peeled Diced	2 x medium (200g/7oz)

Method

1. Heat infused oil in saucepan.
2. Brown diced chicken. Simmer at low heat.
3. Heat margarine in a pot and make a roux with corn flour and a small amount of milk.
4. Add the rest of the milk, stirring regularly to make a smooth sauce.
5. Add ground dried basil.
6. Add to the browned chicken and allow to simmer to cook chicken.
7. When cooked, remove from heat and servings of with mashed potato or steamed rice and low roughage seasonal vegetables

Have a great meal!

Nutritional Analysis Per Serving

USA: Energy (kj/kcal): 2821 (674), Protein (g): 27, Carbohydrate (g): 75, Sugar (g): 3, Total Fat (g): 21, Sodium (mg): 1376, Dietary Fiber (g): 8
Australia: Energy (kj/kcal): 1420 (339) Protein (g): 28, Carbohydrate (g): 20, Sugar (g): 3, Total Fat (g): 21, Sodium (mg): 1376, Dietary Fiber (g): 8
New Zealand: Energy (kj/kcal): 1681 (401), Protein (g): 29, Carbohydrate (g): 22, Sugar (g): 3, Total Fat (g): 22, Sodium (mg): 455 , Dietary Fiber (g): 3

Week 2: Day 6: Spaghetti Bolognaise with Broccoli

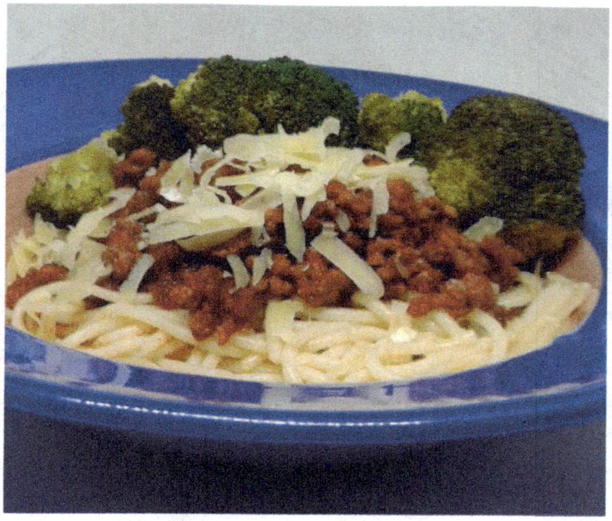

Ingredients	Quantity	Ingredients	Quantity
Tomato Paste	4 Tb	Onion Infused Oil	1 Tb
Beef Mince	220g or 8 oz	Spaghetti, Dried	120g or 4 oz
Ground Cumin Seed	1 Tb	Grated Cheese	40g or 1.5oz
Salt Table	1 dash	Broccoli Floret	2 florets
Garlic infused Oil	1 Tb		

Method

To cook Bolognaise

1. Add the tomato paste into a strainer and remove all seeds and skins etc.
2. Heat garlic infused oil and onion infused oil in a non-stick frying pan.
3. Brown beef mince.
4. Add the crushed tomato liquid and allow to simmer down using low heat.
5. Mix ground cumin.
6. Add salt to taste.
7. Remove from heat.

To cook Spaghetti

1. In a large pan, boil water
2. Add spaghetti to water
3. Boil for 12 minutes.
4. Drain off water.
5. Serve with bolognaise.
6. Add grated cheese on top before serving.

Nutritional Analysis Per Serving

USA: Energy (kj/kcal): 2116 (506), Protein (g): 35, Carbohydrate (g): 36, Sugar (g): 5, Total Fat (g): 23, Sodium (mg): 763, Dietary Fiber (g): 3

Australia: Energy (kj/kcal): 1989 (475) Protein (g): 33, Carbohydrate (g): 71, Sugar (g): 2, Total Fat (g): 18, Sodium (mg): 341, Dietary Fiber (g): 8

New Zealand: Energy (kj/kcal): 2040 (488), Protein (g): 39, Carbohydrate (g): 43, Sugar (g): 3, Total Fat (g): 18, Sodium (mg): 268 , Dietary Fiber (g): 5

Week 2: Day 7: Corned Silverside, Sweet Potato, Carrot, Silverbeet/Swiss Chard

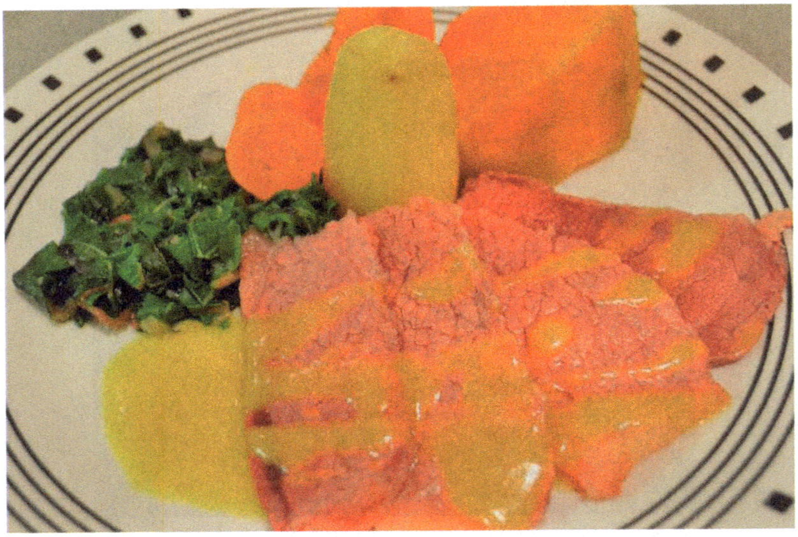

Ingredients	Quantity	Ingredients	Quantity
Corned Silverside	250g / 9 oz	Sweet Potato / Kumara	200g or 7oz
Malt Vinegar	2 Tb	Pumpkin	80g or 3 oz
Bay Leaves	1	Swiss Chard / Silverbeet	80g or 3 oz
Cloves	4	Ready Made – Seedless Mustard Sauce	½ cup
Water	2 cups		

Method

1. In a slow cooker, place corned silverside.
2. Add malt vinegar, cloves, and bay leaf to this.
3. Cover in water.
4. Cook on high for 4 – 6 hours until meat is tender.
5. Remove bay leaf and cloves.
6. Peel and dice pumpkin and kumara.
7. Place in boiling water and cook till soft.
8. When preparing Silverbeet (Swiss chard), just remove the green leaves from white stalk.
9. Boil in water till leaves are soft and cooked.
10. When the corned silverside is ready, slice for service.

Enjoy!

Nutritional Analysis Per Serving

USA: Energy (kj/kcal): 2233 (533), Protein (g): 41, Carbohydrate (g): 40, Sugar (g): 10, Total Fat (g): 18, Sodium (mg): 1483, Dietary Fiber (g): 3

Australia: Energy (kj/kcal): 1360 (325) Protein (g): 23, Carbohydrate (g): 22, Sugar (g): 11, Total Fat (g): 7, Sodium (mg): 814, Dietary Fiber (g): 4

New Zealand: Energy (kj/kcal): 2081 (497), Protein (g): 21, Carbohydrate (g): 64, Sugar (g): 16, Total Fat (g): 18, Sodium (mg): 1799 , Dietary Fiber (g): 4

Week 3: Day 1: Beef Curry, Rice, and Spinach

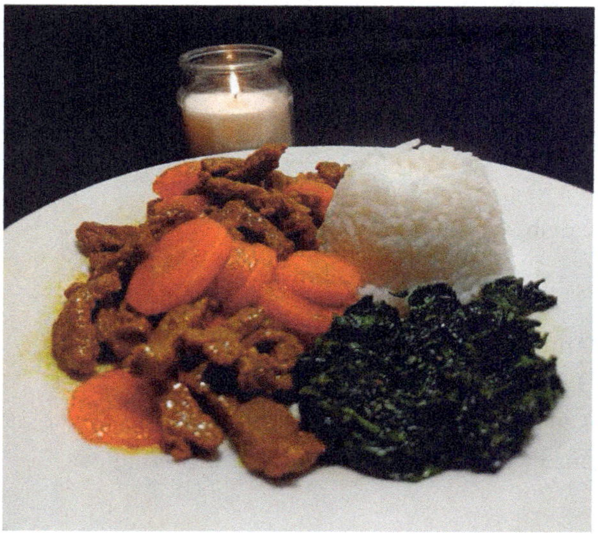

Ingredient	Quantity	Ingredient	Quantity
Olive Oil	7 Tb	Turmeric	1 tsp
Cardamon Pods	2	Beef strips or diced	220g (½ pound)
Cinnamon Stick	3 cm long	Carrot - sliced round	2 large
Coriander Seed	2 Tb	Spinach	12 large leaves
Star Anise	1 flower	Rice	½ cup
Garlic	2 cloves	Onion - fine diced	½ onion
Water	½ cup	Corn flour	1 Tb

Method

In this recipe, I tried a different method to see if I can produce a delicious low roughage beef curry from scratch. It works, deliciously.

To cook the beef curry

1. In a mortar, add garlic, cardamon, cinnamon stick, coriander seeds, star anise. Using mortar, crush into fine powder.
2. In a pot, add 3 Tb of the oil. Sauté onion until it is clear.
3. Add the garlic paste to this. On low heat for a minute, until the garlic looks crisp.
4. Add the 2 Tb of oil to this. Remove from heat.
5. Put another pot on stove, on medium heat.
6. Pour the mixture onto a sieve that is held above the second pot on the stove.
7. Use a teaspoon and press through the oil from the rough fried mixture into the second pot. The oil is now infused with all the spices.
8. Add turmeric to this.
9. Add diced or stripped beef into the second pot. Stir the beef to coat the beef pieces with the spices.

10. Add sliced carrots to this.
11. Add ½ cup water to this and mix through.
12. Allow to simmer on low heat for 10 minutes.
13. When cooked, mix corn flour in couple of tablespoons of curried liquid from the beef curry.
14. Add to the beef curry and simmer further for another 10 minutes to cook the beef and carrot.
15. When cooked, turn off the stove and put aside for service.

Cook rice in the microwave

1. Put rice in microwaveable dish,
2. Wash 3 times.
3. Add 1 cup water to rice.
4. Microwave on high for 10 minutes.
5. Take out and let it sit for 3 minutes.
6. Check that the rice is cooked by pressing a flake in-between your finger and your thumb.

If still uncooked, add a bit more water and cook for further 2-3 minutes.

To light fry the spinach

1. Remove stem from the spinach as discussed in Chapter 4.
2. Slice spinach leaves into thin strips.
3. Heat remaining 2 Tb of oil in a pot.
4. Add sliced spinach to this.
5. Add salt and stir to cook.
6. When spinach has been lightly fried, serve with beef curry and rice.

Like they say in Hindi – Saward! (Delicious!)

Nutritional Analysis Per Serving

USA: Energy (kj/kcal): 3047 (728), Protein (g): 28, Carbohydrate (g): 22, Sugar (g): 5, Total Fat (g): 58, Sodium (mg): 164, Dietary Fiber (g): 7
Australia: Energy (kj/kcal): 2776 (663), Protein (g): 34, Carbohydrate (g): 49, Sugar (g): 6, Total Fat (g): 34, Sodium (mg): 110, Dietary Fiber (g): 10
New Zealand: Energy (kj/kcal): 3555 (850), Protein (g): 29, Carbohydrate (g): 53, Sugar (g): 6, Total Fat (g): 58, Sodium (mg): 102 , Dietary Fiber (g): 8

Week 3: Day 2: Marinated Pork With Flat Bread

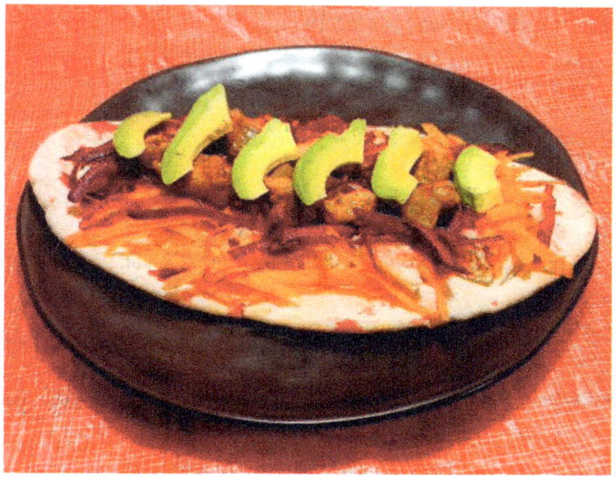

Ingredient	Quantity	Ingredient	Quantity
Garlic - crushed	1 Tb	Pork Sirloin	220g (½ pound)
Soy Sauce - low salt	¼ cup	Cauliflower	½ medium sized
Honey	2 Tb	Carrot (medium size)	2
Ginger - Powder	½ tsp	Avocado	½
Sesame Oil	1 Tb	Flat Bread	2
Salt & Pepper to taste		Beetroot	1
Olive oil	1 Tb x 2		

Method

To prepare pork kebab

1. Cut pork sirloin into 2cm cubes.
2. Prepare soy sauce marinate: in a bowl, add soy sauce, ginger powder, crushed garlic, and honey and mix well.
3. Put the pork sirloin cubes into the marinate, mix through, covering the pork cubes. Leave in covered bowl for 20 minutes.
4. 5. In a frying pan, heat the first tablespoon of oil and cook the pork sirloin (remove the cubed pork sirloin from the rest of the marinate). If the pan is drying out, add a bit more of the marinate into the pan.
6. When cooked, remove cooked pork from heat and put on a clean bowl. Cover this.

To prepare the vegetable fillings

1. Cut the florets of the cauliflower (removing the stems) and divide the florets into smaller florets.
2. Peel and grate the carrot in a bowl. Do the same for the beetroot.
3. Slice avocado into 4-6 slices (depending on the size of the avocado).
4. Heat a wok or skillet. Add some oil to this.
5. Lightly fry the cauliflower florets.
6. Add salt to taste. When cooked, put aside.

Plating

1. Place the flat bread on a plate.

2. Layer cauliflower, beetroot and carrot on it.
3. Place half of the marinated pork on the each flat bread.
5. Lay sliced avocado on the top.

Bona Petitte.

Nutritional Analysis Per Serving

USA: Energy (kj/kcal): 1987 (415), Protein (g): 42, Carbohydrate (g): 28, Sugar (g): 27, Total Fat (g): 19, Sodium (mg): 2122, Dietary Fiber (g): 17

Australia: Energy (kj/kcal): 2796 (604), Protein (g): 39, Carbohydrate (g): 72, Sugar (g): 41, Total Fat (g):23, Sodium (mg): 2001, Dietary Fiber (g): 14

New Zealand: Energy (kj/kcal): 2613 (550), Protein (g): 37, Carbohydrate (g): 71, Sugar (g): 25, Total Fat (g): 21, Sodium (mg): , Dietary Fiber (g): 9

Week 3: Day 3: Chicken Chow Mein

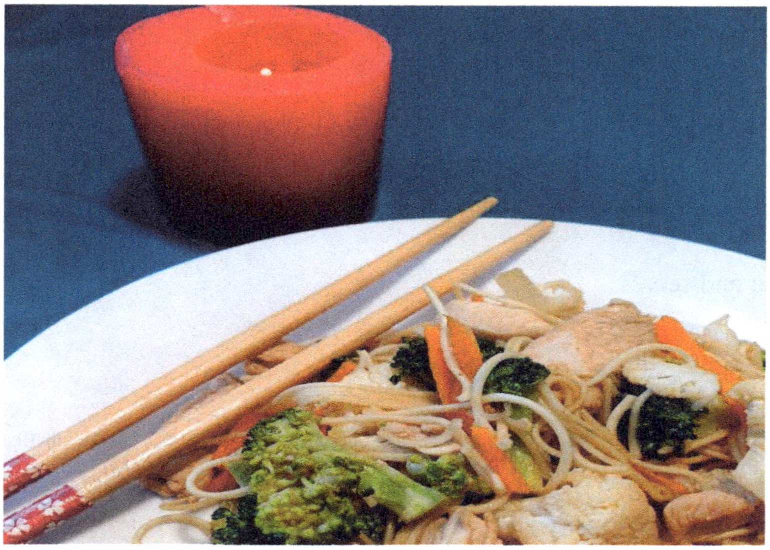

Ingredient	Quantity	Ingredient	Quantity
Chicken Tenderloins or Thigh	200g (6 oz)	Chow Mein Sauce	
Onion Infused Oil	1 Tb	Soy Sauce – low salt	1 ½ Tb
Garlic Infused Oil	1 Tb	Oyster Sauce	1 ½ Tb
Cauliflower	4 florets	Sesame Oil	½ Tb
Carrot (medium size)	2	Corn flour	2 tsp
Broccoli	4 florets	White Pepper	To taste
Chow Mein Noodles	85g (3 oz)	Water	½ cup

Method

Make the sauce

In a bowl, add all the sauce ingredients together and put to side.

Prepare the vegetables

1. Prepare the florets of cauliflower and broccoli: each floret can be cut into 4 slices or you can slice them too.
2. Julienne cut carrots (3 inch in length).

Prepare the chicken & noodles

1. Slice chicken tenderloin or thigh to 3-inch slices. I prefer to use tenderloin or thigh as it is moister compared to the chicken breast which can be dryer.
2. Pour the Chow Mein sauce onto this, mix to coat the chicken and put aside for 10 minutes.
3. In a wok or pan, heat garlic and onion infused oil.
4. Add the marinated chicken meat (not the sauce) to the wok and cook to make a tinged color (but not fully cook).

5. Add the vegetables to this and cook for 2 minutes, stirring occasionally. Vegetables should remain crunchy.
6. Add Chow Mein noodles to the wok.
7. Add the leftover sauce.
8. Stir fry for couple of minutes till the noodles are cooked. Use a pair of tongs to separate the Chow Mein noodles. (Alternatively, you can cook the Chow Mein noodles in a separate pot of boiling water. When cooked au dente, drain out the hot water. Then rinse under cold water. Then add to the chicken vegetable mix above).
9. Remove from heat and serve.

"吃得开心" = Enjoy your meal

Nutritional Analysis Per Serving

USA: Energy (kj/kcal): 2264 (541), Protein (g): 24, Carbohydrate (g): 40, Sugar (g): 5, Total Fat (g): 35, Sodium (mg): 1417, Dietary Fiber (g): 5
Australia: Energy (kj/kcal): 2072 (459), Protein (g): 29, Carbohydrate (g): 50, Sugar (g): 7, Total Fat (g): 18, Sodium (mg): 1386, Dietary Fiber (g): 6
New Zealand: Energy (kj/kcal): 2494 (596), Protein (g): 32, Carbohydrate (g): 72, Sugar (g): 14, Total Fat (g): 20, Sodium (mg): 654 , Dietary Fiber (g): 6

Week 3: Day 4: Beef Casserole

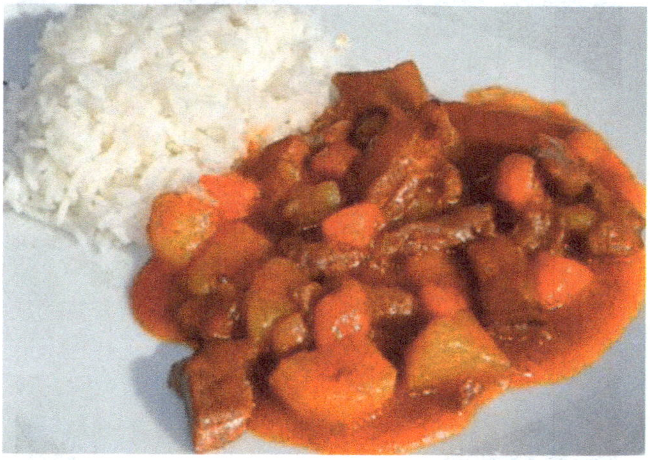

Ingredient	Quantity	Ingredient	Quantity
Garlic Oil	1 Tb	Paprika	1 tsp
Infused Onion Oil	1 Tb	Corn flour	1 Tb
Diced Beef	200g	Carrots diced	1 medium
Water	½ cup	Potatoes, Peeled, Diced	2 (120g/ 4.2 oz
Worcestershire Sauce	2 tsp	Salt, Table	2 dashes
		Rice, Basmati	1 cup

Method

1. Heat garlic infused oil and onion infused oil on a non-stick frying pan.
2. Add diced beef and sauté to seal the meat. Remove from heat.
3. In a crock pot, add all the rest of the ingredients except corn flour. Add sealed diced beef
4. Slow cook for 6 hours.
5. Stir in corn flour in the liquid component.
6. Slow cook for another hour or two.

To cook rice in the microwave

1. Put rice in microwaveable dish,
2. Wash 3 times. Add water to rice. The measurement of water is done like this. Put your pointer finger to the top of the rice. Add water to the first knuckle.
4. Microwave on high for 9 minutes.
5. Take out and let it sit for 3 minutes.
6. Check that rice is cooked by pressing a flake in-between your finger and your thumb.
7. If still uncooked, add a bit more water and cook for further 2-3 minutes.

Let's eat and enjoy!

Nutritional Analysis Per Serving

USA: Energy (kj/kcal): 2062 (493), Protein (g): 26, Carbohydrate (g): 56, Sugar (g): 7, Total Fat (g): 16, Sodium (mg): 416, Dietary Fiber (g): 7

Australia: Energy (kj/kcal): 1632 (309), Protein (g): 27, Carbohydrate (g): 30, Sugar (g): 7, Total Fat (g): 17, Sodium (mg): 771, Dietary Fiber (g): 7

New Zealand: Energy (kj/kcal): 2494 (835), Protein (g): 37, Carbohydrate (g): 110, Sugar (g): 56, Total Fat (g): 27, Sodium (mg): 1346 , Dietary Fiber (g): 3

Week 3: Day 5: Fish Baked In Coconut Cream, Sweet Potato & Spinach

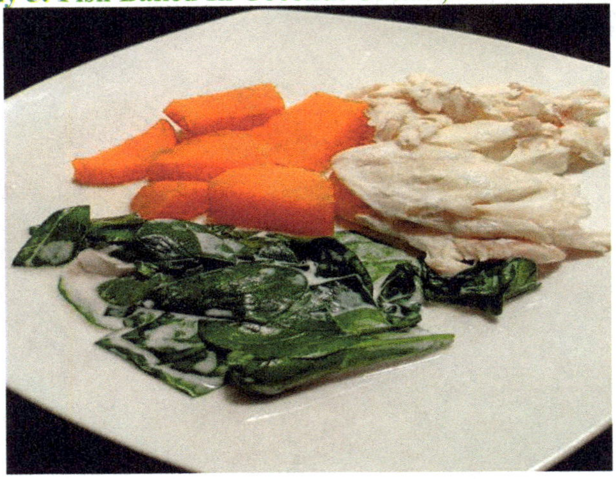

Ingredient	Quantity	Ingredient	Quantity
Fish fillet	200g or 7 oz (2 fillets)	Spinach – baby	3 cups
Garlic - crushed	4 cloves	Sweet Potato	200g or 7 oz
Onion - diced	½ medium	Coconut Cream	200ml or 7oz
Fennel seed - ground	2 Tb	Salt & Pepper to taste	
Olive Oil	3 Tb		

Method:
Heat oven to 180°C / 356°F

Infuse oil

1. In a small pot on stove, heat olive oil.
2. Add diced onion and fry till onion looks clear.
3. Add garlic and ground fennel to this.
4. Allow to fry for couple of minutes until onion turns to light brown color.
5. Remove pot from stove, use a sieve and pour oil through this, separating onion, garlic, and fennel from infused oil.

Prepare fish dish

1. In an oven safe dish, layer fish fillet.
2. Remove stalk from baby spinach leave and discard. Add a layer baby spinach on the fish fillet.
3. Add the infused oil & salt with the coconut cream and mix through.
4. Pour the coconut cream mix on top of the fillet/baby spinach.
5. Cover the dish with aluminum foil and cook for 30 minutes to 35 minutes.
6. Take out of oven and check that the fillet is completely cooked through.
7. If cooked, then serve with the rest of the meal.
8. If fish is not cooked, put back into oven for another 10 minutes.

Boil Sweet Potato

1. Peel the skin off sweet potato.
2. Dice sweet potato into smaller pieces.
3. Place a pot of water on stove to cook sweet kumara in.
4. Add diced sweet potato and boil the water.
5. Turn down the heat, and simmer to cook the sweet potato.
6. Check to see if it is cooked.
7. If cooked, remove from stove for service.

This was a Fiji inspired meal: so **Kakana Vinaka"** roughly translates to "Enjoy your food" or "Enjoy your meal.

Nutritional Analysis Per Serving

USA: Energy (kj/kcal): 1900 (454), Protein (g): 24, Carbohydrate (g): 17, Sugar (g): 5, Total Fat (g): 29, Sodium (mg): 538, Dietary Fiber (g): 6

Australia: Energy (kj/kcal): 1827 (437, Protein (g): 30, Carbohydrate (g): 22, Sugar (g): 7, Total Fat (g): 25, Sodium (mg): 551, Dietary Fiber (g): 5

New Zealand: Energy (kj/kcal): 2443 (584), Protein (g): 31, Carbohydrate (g): 29, Sugar (g): 13, Total Fat (g): 38, Sodium (mg): 507 , Dietary Fiber (g): 9

Week 3: Day 6: Swiss Chard (Silverbeet) Lamb Lasagna

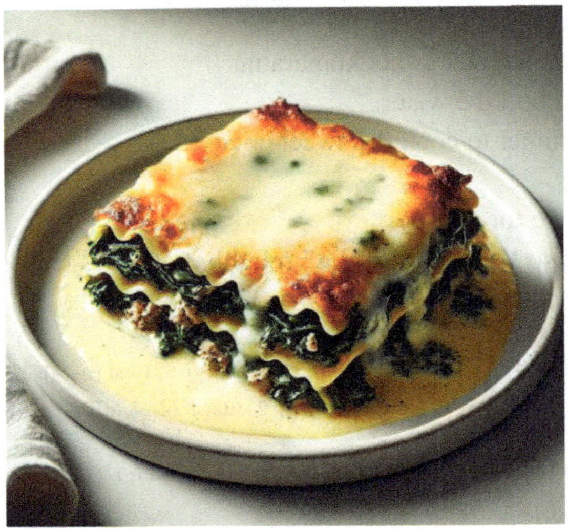

Ingredient	Quantity	Ingredient	Quantity
Garlic Infused Oil	1 Tb	Silverbeet (Swiss Chard)	8 leaves
Onion Infused Oil	1 Tb	Fresh Lasagna sheet	2 sheets
Dried Basil Leaves	1 ½ tsp	Cheese (Cheddar)	½ cup - grated
Fennel seeds	1 tsp	Milk	
Lamb Mince	200g (7 oz)	Milk	2 cups
Tomato Passata Sauce* (strained pureed tomato)	1 cup	Margarine or Butter	2 Tb
		Flour, white	
Salt & Pepper			

In NZ, I found a tomato passata but it still had tomato seeds in it. So, I used a sieve to remove the tomato seeds, before I used the clear passata.

Method

Turn oven to 180°C /350°F

Cook Lamb Mince

1. In very small pot, heat garlic infused oil and garlic infused oil.
2. While this is heating, finely grind fennel seed and dried basil leaves with mortar and pastel.
3. Add to the heated oil. Allow to fry for 30 seconds.
4. Remove from heat, use a sieve to remove the seeds and leaves from the oil. Keep the oil. (alternatively, you can skip the above by using 2 Tb of Italian Infused Oil instead.).
5. Heat a skillet and add the sieved oil or Italian Infused Oil to this.
6. Add lamb mince and brown.
7. When mince has browned, add the tomato passata sauce. Mix well. Allow to simmer for 5 minutes, checking to make sure that the mince thickens. Turn off the heat and set aside.

Prepare Swiss Chard / Silverbeet

As discussed in an earlier section, remove the white stems from the leaves. Discard the stems. Finely chop the green leaves.

Prepare White Sauce

1. In a small pot, heat margarine or butter.
2. Add flour to this to make a paste. Cook for 1 minute.
3. Whisk in milk to this mixture to avoid forming lumps.
4. Add salt & pepper to taste.
5. Add ¾ cup of grated cheese.

Assemble Lasagna

1. Divide the lamb mince, sliced silver beet / Swiss chard and sauce into 2 lots. Lasagna sheets should be for 2 layers.
2. Using a suitable oven safe dish, at the bottom, place half of the lamb mince, then add a layer of sliced Swiss chard / Silverbeet, then layer sheets of lasagna, then add equivalent to half a cup of white sauce.
3. Repeat the same process.
4. After the final layer of lasagna sheet, add grated cheddar cheese on the top.
5. Bake for 30 minutes to 40 minutes till the lasagna is cooked.
6. Remove from oven and serve.

You can make yourself a low roughage salad to go on the side: Baby Spinach Leaves, Cucumber and Carrot with some dressing.
Wishing you a tasty meal!

Nutritional Analysis Per Serving
USA: Energy (kj/kcal): 3868 (925), Protein (g): 40, Carbohydrate (g): 68, Sugar (g): 16, Total Fat (g): 52, Sodium (mg): 1490, Dietary Fiber (g): 11
Australia: Energy (kj/kcal): 3140 (750), Protein (g): 45, Carbohydrate (g): 62, Sugar (g): 19, Total Fat (g): 34, Sodium (mg): 928, Dietary Fiber (g): 9
New Zealand: Energy (kj/kcal): 3581 (856), Protein (g): 45, Carbohydrate (g): 77, Sugar (g): 19, Total Fat (g):41, Sodium (mg): 1043 , Dietary Fiber (g): 7

Week 3: Day 7: Chicken Meatballs with Rice, Broccoli & Cauliflower

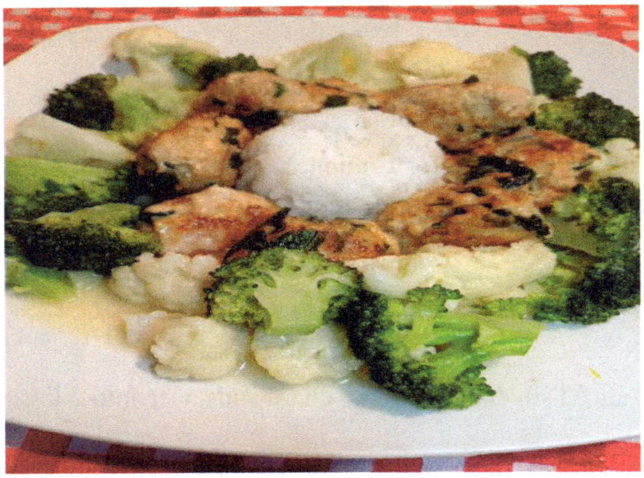

Ingredient	Quantity	Ingredient	Quantity
Garlic Infused Oil	1 Tb	Broccoli	6 florets
Onion Infused Oil	1 Tb	Salt	
Chicken - Minced	220g or 8 oz	Margarine or Butter	2 Tb
Sweet Paprika - ground	1 Tb	Milk	½ cup
Ground Cumin	1 Tb	Flour	4 Tb
Coriander - ground	1 Tb	Parsley	1 bunch
Cauliflower	6 florets	Oil for frying	
Spinach - baby	1 cup	Rice	½ cup

Method

Cook Chicken Meatballs

1. Wash minced chicken and drain.
2. Add paprika, cumin, coriander, salt, flour to the chicken and mix well.
3. Chop spinach leaves into small sizes (after taking off the stalk) add to the mixture above.
4. Add garlic infused oil and onion infused oil to this. Mix well.
5. Roll out chicken meatballs. This will make approximately 14 small meatballs.
6. Heat enough oil in a skillet and fry the meatballs, turning sides to cook all the way through.
7. Once cooked, remove from heat and put aside.

Steam or boil broccoli and cauliflower floret.

1. Prepare the broccoli and cauliflower florets as discussed in chapter 4.
2. Boil in a pot of water. Once the vegetables are cooked to your liking, drain off water and put aside.

Cook rice in the microwave

1. Put rice in microwaveable dish,
2. Wash 3 times.
3. Add 1 cup water to rice.

4. Microwave on high for 10 minutes.
5. Take out and let it sit for 3 minutes.
6. Check that the rice is cooked by pressing a flake in-between your finger and your thumb.
If still uncooked, add a bit more water and cook for further 2-3 minutes.

Prepare Parsley Sauce

1. Chop parsley leaves into small pieces.
2. Add to a pot of milk and simmer for to extract flavors. Add salt to taste.
3. Take the above mix and puree through using a stick blender.
4. Sieve this through into a bowl to remove parsley leaves. Discard the leaves.
5. Heat butter/margarine to melt in a small pot.
6. Add flour to this and make a roux, using a small amount of parsley milk.
7. Add the rest of the parsley milk to this and simmer to thicken sauce.
8. Serve the above components on a plate, pouring parsley sauce on the vegetables and meatballs.

May your taste buds be delighted!

Nutritional Analysis Per Serving

USA: Energy (kj/kcal): 2879 (687), Protein (g): 54, Carbohydrate (g): 34, Sugar (g): 6, Total Fat (g): 36, Sodium (mg): 638, Dietary Fiber (g): 5

Australia: Energy (kj/kcal): 2458 (587), Protein (g): 46, Carbohydrate (g): 49, Sugar (g): 11, Total Fat (g): 5.5, Sodium (mg): 543, Dietary Fiber (g): 7

New Zealand: Energy (kj/kcal): 1978 (473), Protein (g): 34, Carbohydrate (g): 37, Sugar (g): 10, Total Fat (g):21, Sodium (mg): 486 , Dietary Fiber (g): 4

Chapter 13

Country Specific, Gender Specific, Portion Guidelines To Meet Recommended Daily Allowance (USA) or Recommended Dietary Intake (Aust, NZ) For The 21 Day Low Roughage Menu (Phase 2)

Note: Gender is defined in this book as a "Male" or a "Female" for nutritional analysis as RDA / RDI and nutritional analysis programs only use these two terms for their recommendations and analysis.

United States of America Guidelines

To Meet Daily Recommended Dietary Allowance (RDA) For the 21 Days of Low Roughage Diet Menu
(Phase 2)

Calculated for Average Sized Person, Undertaking light activity.

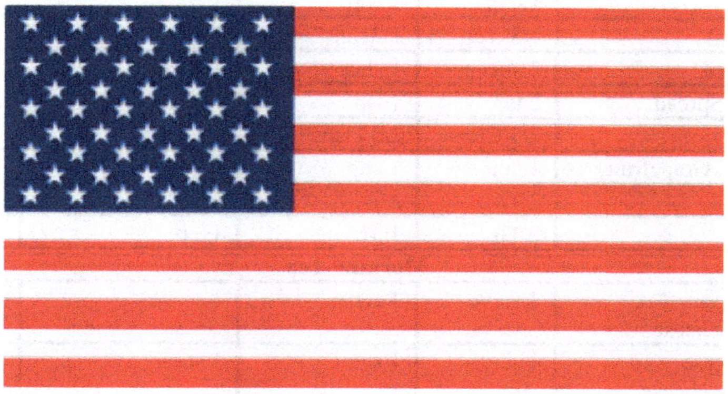

USA Female (Standard)

Age Category (years)	40 -49	50 - 59	60-69	70 -79	80 plus
Breakfast					
Porridge	1 cup	1 cup	1 cup	1 cup	1 cup
Cornflakes	1 cup	1 cup	1 cup	1 cup	1 cup
Ricies	1 cup	1 cup	1 cup	1 cup	1 cup
Stewed fruit (apple, pear, peaches)	1/3 cup	1/3 cup	1/3 cup	1/3 cup	1/3 cup
White Bread or Whole Meal Bread	2 slices	1 slice	1 slice	1 slice	1 slice
Margarine or Butter or Avocado Spread	2 tsp	1 tsp	1 tsp	1 tsp	1 tsp
Milk	2/3 Cup	2/3 Cup	2/3 Cup	2/3 Cup	2/3 Cup
Fruit Juice (clear: Orange, Apple, Grapefruit)	1 cup	1 cup	1 cup	1 cup	1 cup
Peanut Butter	2 Tb	2 Tb	2 Tb	2 Tb	30g
Brown sugar	2 Tb	1 Tb	1 Tb	1 Tb	1 Tb
Morning Tea					
Water Crackers with Cream Cheese: 1 serve = 2 crackers, 1 Tb cream cheese	1 serve	1 serve	1 serve	1 serve	1 serve
Water Crackers with Cottage Cheese 1 serve = 2 crackers, 1 Tb cottage cheese	1 serve	1 serve	1 serve	1 serve	1 serve
Water Crackers with Cheese 1 serve = 2 crackers , 0.7 oz cheese	1 serve	1 serve	1 serve	1 serve	1 serve
Arrowroot Cookies	2	2	2	2	2
Lunch					
Soup	1 cup	1 cup	1 cup	1 cup	1 cup
Protein sandwich (1 serve = 2 slices white bread/ wholemeal bread) with 0.7oz protein	1 serve	1 serve	1 serve	1 serve	1 serve
Afternoon Tea					
Water Crackers with Cream Cheese: 1 serve = 2 crackers, 1 Tb cream cheese	1 serve	1 serve	1 serve	1 serve	1 serve
Water Crackers with Cottage Cheese 1 serve = 2 crackers, 1 Tb cottage cheese	1 serve	1 serve	1 serve	1 serve	1 serve
Water Crackers with Cheese 1 serve = 2 crackers , 0.7 oz cheese	1 serve	1 serve	1 serve	1 serve	1 serve
Arrowroot Cookies	2	2	2	2	2
Soft Banana	1	1	1	1	1
With Hot chocolate	1 cup	1 cup	1 cup	1 cup	1 cup
Dinner					
Protein Component	1 serve	1 serve	1 serve	1 serve	1 serve
Starch Component (potato, rice, kumara, mashed potato etc.)	½ cup (0.4oz)	½ cup or 4 oz	½ cup	½ cup	½ cup
Allowed Low Roughage Vegetables	1/3 cup	1/3 cup	1/3 cup	1/3 cup	1/3 cup
Ice Cream	½ cup	½ cup	½ cup	½ cup	½ cup
Custard	2/3 cup	2/3 cup	2/3 cup	2/3 cup	2/3 cup
Allowed Stewed Fruit	½ cup	½ cup	½ cup	½ cup	½ cup
Supper					
Arrowroot Cookies	2	2	2	2	2
With Milky Drink	1 cup	1 cup	1 cup	1 cup	1 cup

* Milk Drink – Is required twice a day. Similarly, tea, coffees, milo and other fluid are allowed but not needed to meet the recommended daily requirement.
** once a day, ½ Cup of plain yoghurt, can be fruit flavored, no pips or seeds is recommended.

USA Male (Standard)

Age Category (years)	40 -49	50 - 59	60-69	70 -79	80 plus
Breakfast					
Porridge	1 cup	1 cup	1 cup	1 cup	1 cup
Cornflakes	1 cup	1 cup	1 cup	1 cup	1 cup
Ricies	1 cup	1 cup	1 cup	1 cup	1 cup
Stewed fruit (apple, pear, peaches)	1/3 cup	1/3 cup	1/3 cup	1/3 cup	1/3 cup
White Bread or Whole Meal Bread	2 slices	1 slice	1 slice	1 slice	1 slice
Margarine or Butter or Avocado Spread	2 teaspoons	1 teaspoon	1 teaspoon	1 teaspoon	1 teaspoon
Milk	2/3 Cup	2/3 Cup	2/3 Cup	2/3 Cup	2/3 Cup
Fruit Juice (clear: Orange, Apple, Grapefruit)	1 cup	1 cup	1 cup	1 cup	1 cup
Peanut Butter	2 Tb	2 Tb	2 Tb	2 Tb	30g
Brown sugar	2 Tb	1 Tb	1 Tb	1 Tb	1 Tb
Morning Tea					
Water Crackers with Cream Cheese: 1 serve = 2 crackers, 1 Tb cream cheese	2 serves	1 serve	1 serve	1 serve	1 serve
Water Crackers with Cottage Cheese 1 serve = 2 crackers, 1 Tb cottage cheese	2 serves	1 serve	1 serve	1 serve	1 serve
Water Crackers with Cheese 1 serve = 2 crackers , 0.7 oz cheese	2 serves	1 serve	1 serve	1 serve	1 serve
Arrowroot Cookies	4	2	2	2	2
Lunch					
Soup	1 cup	1 cup	1 cup	1 cup	1 cup
Protein sandwich (1 serve = 2 slices white bread/ wholemeal bread) with 20g or 0.7oz protein filling	2 serves	2 serves	2 serves	2 serves	2 serves
Afternoon Tea					
Water Crackers with Cream Cheese: 1 serve = 2 crackers, 1 Tb cream cheese	2 serves	1 serve	1 serve	1 serve	1 serve
Water Crackers with Cottage Cheese 1 serve = 2 crackers, 1 Tb cottage cheese	2 serves	1 serve	1 serve	1 serve	1 serve
Water Crackers with Cheese 1 serve = 2 crackers , 0.7 oz cheese	2 serves	1 serve	1 serve	1 serve	1 serve
Arrowroot Cookies	4	2	2	2	2
Soft Banana	1	1	1	1	1
With Hot chocolate	1 cup	1 cup	1 cup	1 cup	1 cup
Dinner					
Protein Component	1 serve	1 serve	1 serve	1 serve	1 serve
Starch Component (potato, rice, kumara, mashed potato etc.)	½ cup (0.4oz)	½ cup or 4 oz	½ cup	½ cup	½ cup
Allowed Low Roughage Vegetables	1/3 cup	1/3 cup	1/3 cup	1/3 cup	1/3 cup
Ice Cream	½ cup	½ cup	½ cup	½ cup	½ cup
Custard	2/3 cup	2/3 cup	2/3 cup	2/3 cup	2/3 cup
Allowed Stewed Fruit	½ cup	½ cup	½ cup	½ cup	½ cup
Supper					
Arrowroot Cookies	2	2	2	2	2
With Milky Drink	1 cup	1 cup	1 cup	1 cup	1 cup

* Milk Drink – Is required twice a day. Similarly, tea, coffees, milo and other fluid are allowed but not needed to meet the recommended daily requirement.
** once a day, ½ Cup of plain yoghurt, can be fruit flavored, no pips or seeds is recommended.

USA Female (with Diabetes)

Age Category (years)	40 -49	50 - 59	60-69	70 -79	80 plus
Breakfast					
Porridge (cooked)	1 cup	1 cup	1 cup	1 cup	1 cup
Cornflakes	1 cup	1 cup	1 cup	1 cup	1 cup
Ricies	1 cup	1 cup	1 cup	1 cup	1 cup
Stewed fruit (apple, pear, peaches) – sugar free, drained	½ cup	½ cup	1/3 cup	½ cup	½ cup
White Bread or Whole Meal Bread	2 slices	2 slices	1 slice	2 slices	2 slices
Margarine or Butter	2 teaspoons	2 teaspoons	1 teaspoon	2 teaspoons	2 teaspoons
Milk	½ cup	½ cup	½ cup	½ cup	½ cup
Low Calorie, Sugar Free Drink.	2/3 cup	2/3 cup	2/3 cup	2/3 cup	2/3 cup
Peanut Butter	2 Tb	2 Tb	2 Tb	2 Tb	2 Tb
Plain Yoghurt	½ cup	½ cup	½ cup	½ cup	½ cup
Morning Tea					
Plain Water Crackers/ Cream Cheese 1 serve= 2 crackers, 1 Tb Cream Cheese	1 serve	1 serve	1 serve	1 serve	1 serve
Plain Water Crackers/Cottage Cheese 1 serve = 2 crackers, 1 Tb cottage cheese	1 serve	1 serve	1 serve	1 serve	1 serve
Plain Water Crackers, Margarine / Tuna: 1 serve = 2 crackers, margarine, 1 Tb Tuna	1 serve	1 serve	1 serve	1 serve	1 serve
Plain Water Crackers with Cheese 1 serve = 2 crackers, 0.7oz cheese	1 serve	1 serve	1 serve	1 serve	1 serve
Digestive Biscuits	2	2	2	2	2
Milk (3.25% fat)	1 cup	1 cup	1 cup	1 cup	1 cup
Lunch					
Soup	1 cup	1 cup	1 cup	1 cup	1 cup
Protein sandwich (1 serve = 2 slices white bread/ wholemeal bread); 0.7 oz protein	2 serves	1 serve	1 serve	1 serve	1 serve
Afternoon Tea					
Plain Water Crackers/ Cream Cheese 1 serve= 2 crackers, 1 Tb Cream Cheese	1 serve	1 serve	1 serve	1 serve	1 serve
Plain Water Crackers/Cottage Cheese 1 serve = 2 crackers, 1 Tb cottage cheese	1 serve	1 serve	1 serve	1 serve	1 serve
Plain Water Crackers with Cheese 1 serve = 2 crackers, 0.7oz cheese	1 serve	1 serve	1 serve	1 serve	1 serve
Digestive Biscuits	2	2	2	2	2
Dinner					
Protein Component	1 serve	1 serve	1 serve	1 serve	1 serve
Starch Component (potato, rice, kumara, mashed potato etc.)	½ cup or 4 oz	½ cup or 4 oz	½ cup or 4 oz	½ cup or 4 oz	½ cup or 4 oz
Allowed Low Roughage Vegetables	1/3 cup	1/3 cup	1/3 cup	1/3 cup	1/3 cup
Custard – Sugar Free Or Vanilla Pudding – Sugar Free Or Chocolate Pudding – Sugar Free	½ cup	½ cup	½ cup	½ cup	½ cup
Allowed Stewed Fruit, sugar free - drained	½ cup	½ cup	½ cup	½ cup	½ cup
Sugar Free Jelly Dessert	½ cup	½ cup	½ cup	½ cup	½ cup
Supper					
Plain Water Crackers/ Cream Cheese 1 serve= 2 crackers, 1 Tb Cream Cheese	1 serve	1 serve	1 serve	1 serve	1 serve
Plain Water Crackers/Cottage Cheese 1 serve = 2 crackers, 1 Tb cottage cheese	1 serve	1 serve	1 serve	1 serve	1 serve
Plain Water Crackers with Cheese 1 serve = 2 crackers, 0.7oz cheese	1 serve	1 serve	1 serve	1 serve	1 serve
With Milk (Standard)	1 cup	2	2	2	2
Digestive Biscuits	2	1 cup	1 cup	1 cup	1 cup
** once a day, 125g or ½ Cup of plain yoghurt					

USA Male (with Diabetes)

Age Category (years)	40 -49	50 - 59	60-69	70 -79	80 plus
Breakfast					
Porridge (cooked)	1 cup	1 cup	1 cup	1 cup	1 cup
Cornflakes	1 cup	1 cup	1 cup	1 cup	1 cup
Ricies	1 cup	1 cup	1 cup	1 cup	1 cup
Stewed fruit (apple, pear, peaches) – sugar free, drained	½ cup	1/3 cup	1/3 cup	1/3 cup	1/3 cup
White Bread or Whole Meal Bread	2 slices	2 slices	1 slice	1 slice	1 slice
Margarine or Butter	2 tsp	2 tsp	1 tsp	1 tsp	1 tsp
Milk	½ cup	½ cup	½ cup	½ cup	½ cup
Low Calorie, Sugar Free Drink (Juice or Tea or Coffee etc.).	2/3 cup	2/3 cup	2/3 cup	2/3 cup	2/3 cup
Peanut Butter	2 Tb	2 Tb	2 Tb	2 Tb	2 Tb
Plain Yoghurt	½ cup	½ cup	½ cup	½ cup	½ cup
Morning Tea					
Plain Water Crackers with Cream Cheese: 1 serve = 2 crackers, 1 Tb cream cheese	2 serves	2 serves	1 serve	1 serve	1 serve
Plain Water Crackers with Cottage Cheese : 1 serve = 2 crackers, 1 Tb cottage cheese	2 serves	2 serves	1 serve	1 serve	1 serve
Plain Water Crackers, Margarine with Tuna 1 serve = 2 crackers, 1 tsp margarine, 1 Tb Tuna	2 serves	2 serves	1 serve	1 serve	1 serve
Plain Water Crackers with Cheese: 1 serve = 2 crackers, 0.7oz cheese	2 serves	2 serves	1 serve	1 serve	1 serve
Digestive Biscuits With	4	4	2	2	2
Milk (3.25% fat)	1 cup	1 cup	1 cup	1 cup	1 cup
Lunch					
Soup	1 cup	1 cup	1 cup	1 cup	1 cup
Protein sandwich (1 serve = 2 slices white bread/ wholemeal bread) with 20g or 0.7 oz protein filling	2 serves	2 serves	2 serves	2 serve	2 serves
Afternoon Tea					
Water Crackers with Cream Cheese: 1 serve = 2 crackers, 1 Tb cream cheese	2 serves	2 serves	2 serves	1 serve	1 serve
Plain Water Crackers with Cottage Cheese : 1 serve = 2 crackers, 1 Tb cottage cheese	2 serves	2 serves	2 serves	1 serve	1 serve
Plain Water Crackers with Cheese: 1 serve = 2 crackers, 0.7oz cheese	2 serves	2 serves	2 serves	1 serve	1 serve
Digestive Biscuits	4	4	4	2	2
Dinner					
Protein Component	1 serve	1 serve	1 serve	1 serve	1 serve
Starch Component (potato, rice, kumara, mashed potato etc.)	½ cup or 4 oz	½ cup or 4 oz	½ cup or 4 oz	½ cup or 4 oz	½ cup or 4 oz
Allowed Low Roughage Vegetables	1/3 cup	1/3 cup	1/3 cup	1/3 cup	1/3 cup
Custard – Sugar Free Or Vanilla Pudding – Sugar Free Or Chocolate Pudding – Sugar Free	½ cup	½ cup	½ cup	½ cup	½ cup
Allowed Stewed Fruit, sugar free - drained	½ cup	½ cup	½ cup	½ cup	½ cup
Sugar Free Jelly Dessert	½ cup	½ cup	½ cup	½ cup	½ cup
Supper					
Water Crackers with Cream Cheese: 1 serve = 2 crackers, 1 Tb cream cheese	2 serves	2 serves	2 serves	1 serve	1 serve
Plain Water Crackers with Cottage Cheese : 1 serve = 2 crackers, 1 Tb cottage cheese	2 serves	2 serves	2 serves	1 serve	1 serve
Plain Water Crackers with Cheese: 1 serve = 2 crackers, 0.7oz cheese	2 serves	2 serves	2 serves	1 serve	1 serve
With Milk (Standard)	1 cup	1 cup	1 cup	1 cup	1 cup
Digestive Biscuits	4	4	4	2	2
** once a day, 125g or ½ Cup of plain yoghurt					

New Zealand Guidelines

To Meet Daily Recommended Dietary Intake (RDI) For The 21 Days of Low Roughage Diet Menu (Phase 2)

Calculated for Average Sized Person, Undertaking light activity.

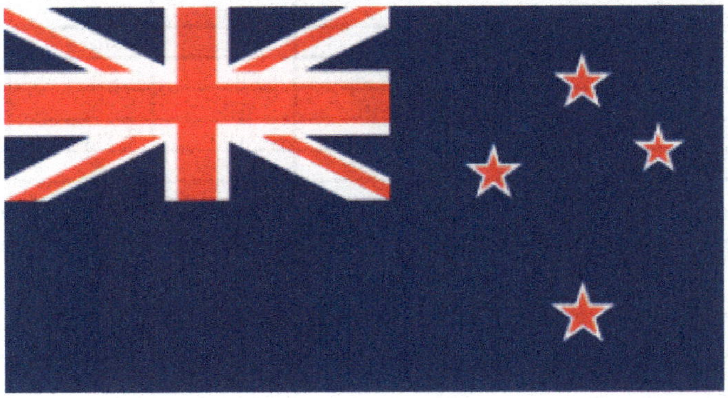

NZ Female (Standard)

Age Category	40 – 49	50 – 59	60 – 69	70 – 79	80+
Breakfast					
Porridge	1 cup	1 cup	1 cup	1 cup	1 cup
Cornflakes	1 cup	1 cup	1 cup	1 cup	1 cup
Rice bubbles	1 cup	1 cup	1 cup	1 cup	1 cup
Stewed fruit (apple, pear, peaches)	1/3 cup	1/3 cup	1/3 cup	1/3 cup	1/3 cup
White Bread or Whole Meal Bread	2 slices	2 slices	2 slice	2 slice	2 slice
Plant Based Spread, Butter or Avocado Spread	2 tsp	2 tsp	2 tsp	2 tsp	2 tsp
Milk	½ cup	½ cup	½ cup	½ cup	½ cup
Fruit Juice (clear: Orange, Apple, Grapefruit)	¾ cup	¾ cup	¾ cup	¾ cup	¾ cup
Peanut Butter	2 Tb	2 Tb	2 Tb	2 Tb	2 Tb
Brown sugar	1 Tb	1 Tb	1 Tb	1 Tb	1 Tb
Morning Tea					
Water Crackers with Cream Cheese: 1 serve = 2 crackers, 1 Tb cream cheese	1 serve	1 serve	1 serve	1 serve	1 serve
Water Crackers with Cottage Cheese: 1 serve = 2 crackers, 1 Tb cottage cheese	1 serve	1 serve	1 serve	1 serve	1 serve
Water Crackers with Cheese: 1 serve = 2 crackers, 20g cheese	1 serve	1 serve	1 serve	1 serve	1 serve
Arrowroot Cookies	4	2	2	2	2
Lunch					
Soup	1 cup	1 cup	1 cup	1 cup	1 cup
Protein sandwich (1 serve = 2 slices white bread/ wholemeal bread) with 20g protein filling	2 serves	1 serve	1 serve	1 serve	1 serve
Banana	1 medium	1 medium	1 medium	1 medium	1 medium
Afternoon Tea					
Water Crackers with Cream Cheese: 1 serve = 2 crackers, 1 Tb cream cheese	1 serve	1 serve	1 serve	1 serve	1 serve
Water Crackers with Cottage Cheese: 1 serve = 2 crackers, 1 Tb cottage cheese	1 serve	1 serve	1 serve	1 serve	1 serve
Water Crackers with Cheese: 1 serve = 2 crackers, 20g cheese	1 serve	1 serve	1 serve	1 serve	1 serve
Fruit Flavored Yoghurt	½ cup	½ cup	½ cup	½ cup	½ cup
Arrowroot Cookies	4	2	2	2	2
Dinner					
Protein Component	1 serve	1 serve	1 serve	1 serve	1 serve
Starch Component (potato, rice, kumara, mashed potato etc.)	½ cup	½ cup	½ cup	½ cup	½ cup
Allowed Low Roughage Vegetables	1/3 cup	1/3 cup	1/3 cup	1/3 cup	1/3 cup
Ice Cream	½ cup	½ cup	½ cup	½ cup	½ cup
Custard	½ cup	½ cup	½ cup	½ cup	½ cup
Allowed Stewed Fruit	1/2 cup	1/2 cup	1/2 cup	1/2 cup	1/2 cup
Age Category	**40 – 49**	**50 – 59**	**60 – 69**	**70 – 79**	**80+**
Supper					
Arrowroot Cookies	4	2	2	2	2

* Milk Drink – Is required twice a day. Similarly, tea, coffees, milo and other fluid are allowed but not needed to meet the recommended daily requirement.
** once a day, ½ Cup of plain yoghurt, can be fruit flavored, no pips or seeds is recommended

NZ Male (Standard)

Age Category	40 – 49	50 – 59	60 – 69	70 – 79	80+
Breakfast					
Porridge	1 cup	1 cup	1 cup	1 cup	1 cup
Cornflakes	1 cup	1 cup	1 cup	1 cup	1 cup
Rice bubbles	1 cup	1 cup	1 cup	1 cup	1 cup
Stewed fruit (apple, pear, peaches)	1/3 cup	1/3 cup	1/3 cup	1/3 cup	1/3 cup
White Bread or Whole Meal Bread	2 slices	1 slice	1 slice	1 slice	1 slice
Plant Based Spread, Butter or Avocado Spread	2 teaspoons	1 teaspoon	1 teaspoon	1 teaspoon	1 teaspoon
Milk	2/3 Cup	2/3 Cup	2/3 Cup	2/3 Cup	2/3 Cup
Fruit Juice (clear: Orange, Apple, Grapefruit)	1 cup	1 cup	1 cup	1 cup	1 cup
Peanut Butter	2 Tb	2 Tb	2 Tb	2 Tb	2 Tb
Brown sugar	2 Tb	1 Tb	1 Tb	1 Tb	1 Tb
Morning Tea					
Water Crackers with Cream Cheese: 1 serve = 2 crackers, 1 Tb cream cheese	1 serve	1 serve	1 serve	1 serve	1 serve
Water Crackers with Cottage Cheese: 1 serve = 2 crackers, 1 Tb cottage cheese	1 serve	1 serve	1 serve	1 serve	1 serve
Water Crackers with Cheese: 1 serve = 2 crackers, 20g cheese	1 serve	1 serve	1 serve	1 serve	1 serve
Arrowroot Cookies	4	2	2	2	2
Lunch					
Soup	1 cup	1 cup	1 cup	1 cup	1 cup
Protein sandwich (1 serve = 2 slices white bread/ wholemeal bread) with 20g protein filling	2 serves	2 serves	2 serves	2 serves	2 serves
Afternoon Tea					
Water Crackers with Cream Cheese: 1 serve = 2 crackers, 1 Tb cream cheese	1 serve	1 serve	1 serve	1 serve	1 serve
Water Crackers with Cottage Cheese: 1 serve = 2 crackers, 1 Tb cottage cheese	1 serve	1 serve	1 serve	1 serve	1 serve
Water Crackers with Cheese: 1 serve = 2 crackers, 20g cheese	1 serve	1 serve	1 serve	1 serve	1 serve
Arrowroot Cookies	4	2	2	½ cup	2
Soft Banana	1	1	1	2	1
With Hot chocolate	1 cup	1 cup	1 cup	1 cup	1 cup
Dinner					
Protein Component	1 serve	1 serve	1 serve	1 serve	1 serve
Starch Component (potato, rice, kumara, mashed potato etc.)	½ cup	½ cup	½ cup	½ cup	½ cup
Allowed Low Roughage Vegetables	1/3 cup	1/3 cup	1/3 cup	1/3 cup	1/3 cup
Ice Cream	½ cup	½ cup	½ cup	½ cup	½ cup
Custard	2/3 cup	2/3 cup	2/3 cup	2/3 cup	½ cup
Allowed Stewed Fruit	½ cup	½ cup	½ cup	½ cup	1/2 cup
Supper					
Arrowroot Cookies	2	2	2	2	2
With Milky Drink	1 cup	1 cup	1 cup	1 cup	1 cup

* Milky Drink – Is required twice a day. Similarly, tea, coffees, milo and other fluid are allowed but not needed to meet the recommended daily requirement.
** once a day, ½ cup of plain yoghurt, can be fruit flavored, no pips or seeds is recommended.

NZ Female (with Diabetes)

Age Category	40 – 49	50 – 59	60 – 69	70 – 79	80 +
Breakfast					
Porridge (cooked)	1 cup	1 cup	1 cup	1 cup	1 cup
Cornflakes	1 cup	1 cup	1 cup	1 cup	1 cup
Rice bubbles	1 cup	1 cup	1 cup	1 cup	1 cup
Stewed fruit (apple, pear, peaches) – sugar free, drained	½ cup	½ cup	1/3 cup	½ cup	½ cup
White Bread or Whole Meal Bread	2 slices	2 slices	1 slices	2 slices	2 slices
Plant Based Spread, Butter or Avocado Spread	2 tsp	2 tsp	1 tsp	2 tsp	2 tsp
Milk	½ cup	½ cup	½ cup	½ cup	½ cup
Low Calorie, Sugar Free Drink (Juice or Tea or Coffee etc.).	2/3 cup	2/3 cup	2/3 cup	2/3 cup	2/3 cup
Peanut Butter	2 Tb	2 Tb	2 Tb	2 Tb	2 Tb
Plain Yoghurt	½ cup	½ cup	½ cup	½ cup	½ cup
Morning Tea					
Plain Water Crackers with Cream Cheese: 1 serve = 2 crackers, 1 Tb cream cheese	1 serve	1 serve	1 serve	1 serve	1 serve
Plain Water Crackers with Cottage Cheese: 1 serve = 2 crackers, 1 Tb cottage cheese	1 serve	1 serve	1 serve	1 serve	1 serve
Plain Water Crackers, with Tuna: 1 serve = 2 crackers, 1 Tb Tuna	1 serve	1 serve	1 serve	1 serve	1 serve
Plain Water Crackers with Cheese: 1 serve = 2 crackers, 20 g Cheese	1 serve	1 serve	1 serve	1 serve	1 serve
Digestive Biscuits With	2	2	2	2	2
Milk (3.25% fat)	1 cup	1 cup	1 cup	1 cup	1 cup
Lunch					
Soup	1 cup	1 cup	1 cup	1 cup	1 cup
Protein sandwich (1 serve = 2 slices white bread/ wholemeal bread) with 30g protein filling	2 serves	1 serve	1 serve	1 serve	1 serve
Afternoon Tea					
Plain Water Crackers with Cream Cheese: 1 serve = 2 crackers, 1 Tb cream cheese	1 serve	1 serve	1 serve	1 serve	1 serve
Plain Water Crackers with Cottage Cheese: 1 serve = 2 crackers, 1 Tb cottage cheese	1 serve	1 serve	1 serve	1 serve	1 serve
Plain Water Crackers, with Tuna: 1 serve = 2 crackers, 1 Tb Tuna	1 serve	1 serve	1 serve	1 serve	1 serve
Digestive Biscuits	2	2	2	2	2
Dinner					
Protein Component	1 serve	1 serve	1 serve	1 serve	1 serve
Starch Component (potato, rice, kumara, mashed potato etc.)	½ cup	½ cup	½ cup	½ cup	½ cup
Allowed Low Roughage Vegetables	1/3 cup	1/3 cup	1/3 cup	1/3 cup	1/3 cup
Custard – Sugar Free Or Vanilla Pudding – Sugar Free Or Chocolate Pudding – Sugar Free	½ cup	½ cup	½ cup	½ cup	½ cup
Allowed Stewed Fruit, sugar free – drained	½ cup	½ cup	½ cup	½ cup	½ cup
Sugar Free Jelly Dessert	½ cup	½ cup	½ cup	½ cup	½ cup
Supper					
Plain Water Crackers with Cream Cheese: 1 serve = 2 crackers, 1 Tb cream cheese	1 serve	1 serve	1 serve	1 serve	1 serve
Plain Water Crackers with Cottage Cheese: 1 serve = 2 crackers, 1 Tb cottage cheese	1 serve	1 serve	1 serve	1 serve	1 serve
Plain Water Crackers with Cheese: 1 serve = 2 crackers, 20 g Cheese	1 serve	1 serve	1 serve	1 serve	1 serve
With Milk (Standard)	1 cup	2	2	2	2
Digestive Biscuits	2	1 cup	1 cup	1	1 cup
* Once a day, 125g or ½ Cup of plain yoghurt					

NZ Male (with Diabetes)

Age Category	40 -49	50 – 59	60 – 69	70 – 79	80+
Breakfast					
Porridge	1 cup	1 cup	1 cup	1 cup	1 cup
Cornflakes	1 cup	1 cup	1 cup	1 cup	1 cup
Rice bubbles	1 cup	1 cup	1 cup	1 cup	1 cup
Stewed fruit (apple, pear, peaches) – sugar free, drained	½ cup	1/3 cup	1/3 cup	1/3 cup	1/3 cup
White Bread or Whole Meal Bread	2 slices	2 slices	1 slice	1 slice	1 slice
Plant Based Spread, Butter or Avocado Spread	2 tsp	2 tsp	1 tsp	1 tsp	1 tsp
Milk	½ cup	½ cup	½ cup	½ cup	½ cup
Low Calorie, Sugar Free Drink (Juice or Tea or Coffee etc.).	2/3 cup	2/3 cup	2/3 cup	2/3 cup	2/3 cup
Peanut Butter	2 Tb	2 Tb	2 Tb	2 Tb	2 Tb
Plain Yoghurt	½ cup	½ cup	½ cup	½ cup	½ cup
Morning Tea					
Plain Water Crackers with Cream Cheese: 1 serve = 2 crackers, 1 Tb cream cheese	1 serve	1 serve	1 serve	1 serve	1 serve
Plain Water Crackers with Cottage Cheese: 1 serve = 2 crackers, 1 Tb cottage cheese	1 serve	1 serve	1 serve	1 serve	1 serve
Plain Water Crackers, with Tuna: 1 serve = 2 crackers, 1 Tb Tuna	1 serve	1 serve	1 serve	1 serve	1 serve
Plain Water Crackers with Cheese: 1 serve = 2 crackers, 20 g Cheese	1 serve	1 serve	1 serve	1 serve	1 serve
Digestive Biscuits	4	4	2	2	2
With Milk (3.25% fat)	1 cup	1 cup	1 cup	1 cup	1 cup
Lunch					
Soup	1 cup	1 cup	1 cup	1 cup	1 cup
Protein sandwich (1 serve = 2 slices white bread/ wholemeal bread) with 1 oz protein filling	2 serves	2 serves	2 serves	2 serves	2 serves
Afternoon Tea					
Plain Water Crackers with Cream Cheese: 1 serve = 2 crackers, 1 Tb cream cheese	1 serve	1 serve	1 serve	1 serve	1 serve
Plain Water Crackers with Cottage Cheese: 1 serve = 2 crackers, 1 Tb cottage cheese	1 serve	1 serve	1 serve	1 serve	1 serve
Plain Water Crackers with Cheese: 1 serve = 2 crackers, 20 g Cheese	1 serve	1 serve	1 serve	1 serve	1 serve
Digestive Biscuits	4	4	4	2	2
Dinner					
Protein Component	1 serve	1 serve	1 serve	1 serve	1 serve
Starch Component (potato, rice, kumara, mashed potato etc.)	½ cup	½ cup	½ cup	½ cup	½ cup
Allowed Low Roughage Vegetables	1/3 cup	1/3 cup	1/3 cup	1/3 cup	1/3 cup
Custard – Sugar Free or Vanilla Pudding – Sugar Free or Sugar Free Chocolate Pudding	½ cup	½ cup	½ cup	½ cup	½ cup
Allowed Stewed Fruit, sugar free – drained	½ cup	½ cup	½ cup	½ cup	½ cup
Sugar Free Jelly	½ cup	½ cup	½ cup	½ cup	½ cup
Supper					
Plain Water Crackers with Cream Cheese: 1 serve = 2 crackers, 1 Tb cream cheese	1 serve	1 serve	1 serve	1 serve	1 serve
Plain Water Crackers with Cottage Cheese: 1 serve = 2 crackers, 1 Tb cottage cheese	1 serve	1 serve	1 serve	1 serve	1 serve
Plain Water Crackers with Cheese: 1 serve = 2 crackers, 20 g Cheese	1 serve	1 serve	1 serve	1 serve	1 serve
With Milk (3.25% fat)	1 cup	1 cup	1 cup	1 cup	1 cup
Digestive Biscuits	4	4	4	2	2
*Once a day, 125g of plain yoghurt					

Australian Guidelines

To Meet Daily Recommended Dietary Intake For The 21 Day Low Roughage Diet Menu (Phase 2)

Calculated for Average Sized Person, Undertaking light activity.

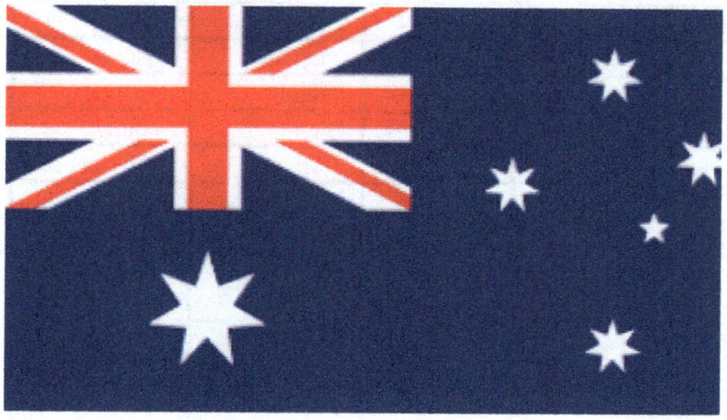

Australian Female (Standard)

Age Categories	40 – 49	50 – 59	60 – 69	70 -79	80 +
Breakfast					
Porridge	1 cup	1 cup	1 cup	1 cup	1 cup
Cornflakes	1 cup	1 cup	1 cup	1 cup	1 cup
Ricies	1 cup	1 cup	1 cup	1 cup	1 cup
Stewed fruit (apple, pear, peaches)	1/3 cup	1/3 cup	1/3 cup	1/3 cup	1/3 cup
White Bread or Whole Meal Bread	2 slices	2 slices	2 slices	2 slices	2 slice
Plant Based Spread, Butter or Avocado Spread	2 tsp	2 tsp	2 tsp	2 tsp	2 tsp
Milk	½ cup	½ cup	½ cup	½ cup	½ cup
Fruit Juice (clear: Orange, Apple, Grapefruit)	¾ cup	¾ cup	¾ cup	¾ cup	¾ cup
Peanut Butter	2 Tb	2 Tb	2 Tb	2 Tb	2 Tb
Brown sugar	1 Tb	1 Tb	1 Tb	1 Tb	1 Tb
Morning Tea					
Water Crackers with Cream Cheese: 1 serve = 2 crackers, 1 Tb cream cheese	1 serve	1 serve	1 serve	1 serve	1 serve
Water Crackers with Cottage Cheese: 1 serve = 2 crackers, 1 Tb cottage cheese	1 serve	1 serve	1 serve	1 serve	1 serve
Water Crackers with Cheese: 1 serve = 2 crackers, 20g cheese	1 serve	1 serve	1 serve	1 serve	1 serve
Arrowroot Cookies	4	2	2	2	2
Lunch					
Soup	1 cup	1 cup	1 cup	1 cup	1 cup
Protein sandwich (1 serve = 2 slices white bread/ wholemeal bread) with 20g protein filling	2 serves	1 serve	1 serve	1 serve	1 serve
Banana	1 medium	1 medium	1 medium	1 medium	1 medium
Afternoon Tea					
Water Crackers with Cream Cheese: 1 serve = 2 crackers, 1 Tb cream cheese	1 serve	1 serve	1 serve	1 serve	1 serve
Water Crackers with Cottage Cheese: 1 serve = 2 crackers, 1 Tb cottage cheese	1 serve	1 serve	1 serve	1 serve	1 serve
Water Crackers with Cheese: 1 serve = 2 crackers, 20g cheese	1 serve	1 serve	1 serve	1 serve	1 serve
Fruit Flavored Yoghurt	½ cup	½ cup	½ cup	½ cup	½ cup
Arrowroot Cookies	4	2	2	2	2
Dinner					
Protein Component	1 serve	1 serve	1 serve	1 serve	1 serve
Starch Component (potato, rice, kumara, mashed potato etc.)	½ cup	½ cup	½ cup	½ cup	½ cup
Allowed Low Roughage Vegetables	1/3 cup	1/3 cup	1/3 cup	1/3 cup	1/3 cup
Ice Cream	½ cup	½ cup	½ cup	½ cup	½ cup
Custard	½ cup	½ cup	½ cup	½ cup	½ cup
Allowed Stewed Fruit	1/2 cup	1/2 cup	1/2 cup	1/2 cup	1/2 cup
Supper					
Arrowroot Cookies	4	2	2	2	2

* Milk Drink – Is required twice a day. Similarly, tea, coffees, milo and other fluid are allowed but not needed to meet the recommended daily requirement.
** Once a day, ½ Cup of plain yoghurt, can be fruit flavored, no pips or seeds is recommended.

Australian Male (Standard)

Age Category	40 -49	50 – 59	60 – 69	70 – 79	80 +
Breakfast					
Porridge	1 cup	1 cup	1 cup	1 cup	1 cup
Cornflakes	1 cup	1 cup	1 cup	1 cup	1 cup
Ricies	1 cup	1 cup	1 cup	1 cup	1 cup
Stewed fruit (apple, pear, peaches)	1/3 cup	1/3 cup	80g	1/3 cup	1/3 cup
White Bread or Whole Meal Bread	2 slices	1 slice	1 slice	1 slice	1 slice
Plant Based Spread, Butter or Avocado Spread	2 tsp	1 tsp	1 tsp	1 tsp	1 tsp
Milk or Plain or Fruit Flavored Yoghurt	2/3 Cup	2/3 Cup	2/3 Cup	2/3 Cup	2/3 Cup
Fruit Juice (clear: Orange, Apple, Grapefruit)	1 cup	1 cup	1 cup	1 cup	1 cup
Cream	2 Tb	2 Tb	30g	2 Tb	30g
Peanut Butter	2 Tb	1 Tb	1 Tb	1 Tb	1 Tb
Morning Tea					
Water Crackers with Cream Cheese: 1 serve = 2 crackers, 1 Tb cream cheese	1 serve	1 serve	1 serve	1 serve	1 serve
Water Crackers with Cottage Cheese: 1 serve = 2 crackers, 1 Tb cottage cheese	1 serve	1 serve	1 serve	1 serve	1 serve
Water Crackers with Cheese: 1 serve = 2 crackers, 20g cheese	1 serve	1 serve	1 serve	1 serve	1 serve
Arrowroot Cookies	4	2	2	2	2
Lunch					
Soup	1 cup	1 cup	1 cup	1 cup	1 cup
Protein sandwich (1 serve = 2 slices white bread/ wholemeal bread) with 20g protein filling	2 serves	2 serves	2 serves	2 serves	2 serves
Age Categories	**40 -49**	**50 -59**	**60 – 69**	**70 – 79**	**80 +**
Afternoon Tea					
Water Crackers with Cream Cheese: 1 serve = 2 crackers, 1 Tb cream cheese	1 serve	1 serve	1 serve	1 serve	1 serve
Water Crackers with Cottage Cheese: 1 serve = 2 crackers, 1 Tb cottage cheese	1 serve	1 serve	1 serve	1 serve	1 serve
Water Crackers with Cheese: 1 serve = 2 crackers, 20g cheese	1 serve	1 serve	1 serve	1 serve	1 serve
Arrowroot Cookies	4	2	2	2	2
Soft Banana	1	1	1	1	1
With Hot chocolate	1 cup	1 cup	1 cup	1 cup	1 cup
Dinner					
Protein Component	1 serve	1 serve	1 serve	1 serve	1 serve
Starch Component (potato, rice, kumara, mashed potato etc.)	½ cup	½ cup	½ cup	½ cup	½ cup
Allowed Low Roughage Vegetables	1/3 cup	1/3 cup	1/3 cup	1/3 cup	1/3 cup
Ice Cream	½ cup	½ cup	½ cup	½ cup	½ cup
Custard	2/3 cup	2/3 cup	2/3 cup	2/3 cup	2/3 cup
Allowed Stewed Fruit	½ cup	½ cup	½ cup	½ cup	½ cup
Supper					
Arrowroot Cookies	2	2	2	2	2
With Milky Drink	1 cup	1 cup	1 cup	1 cup	1 cup

* Milky Drink – Is required twice a day. Similarly, tea, coffees, milo and other fluid are allowed but not needed to meet the recommended daily requirement.
** Once a day, ½ cup of plain yoghurt, can be fruit flavored, no pips or seeds is recommended.

Australian Female (with Diabetes)

Age Categories	40 – 49	50 – 59	60 – 69	70 – 79	80 +
Breakfast					
Porridge (cooked)	1 cup	1 cup	1 cup	1 cup	1 cup
Cornflakes	1 cup	1 cup	1 cup	1 cup	1 cup
Ricies	1 cup	1 cup	1 cup	1 cup	1 cup
Stewed fruit (apple, pear, peaches) – sugar free, drained	½ cup	½ cup	1/3 cup	½ cup	½ cup
White Bread or Whole Meal Bread	2 slices	2 slices	1 slices	2 slices	2 slices
Margarine, Butter or Avocado Spread	2 tsp	2 tsp	2 tsp	2 tsp	2 tsp
Milk	½ cup	½ cup	½ cup	½ cup	½ cup
Low Calorie, Sugar Free Drink (Juice or Tea or Coffee etc.).	2/3 cup	2/3 cup	2/3 cup	2/3 cup	2/3 cup
Peanut Butter	2 Tb	2 Tb	2 Tb	2 Tb	2 Tb
Plain Yoghurt	½ cup	½ cup	½ cup	½ cup	½ cup
Morning Tea					
Plain Water Crackers with Cream Cheese: 1 serve = 2 crackers, 1 Tb cream cheese	1 serve	1 serve	1 serve	1 serve	1 serve
Plain Water Crackers with Cottage Cheese: 1 serve = 2 crackers, 1 Tb cottage cheese	1 serve	1 serve	1 serve	1 serve	1 serve
Plain Water Crackers, with Tuna: 1 serve = 2 crackers, 1 Tb Tuna	1 serve	1 serve	1 serve	1 serve	1 serve
Plain Water Crackers with Cheese: 1 serve = 2 crackers, 20g cheese	1 serve	1 serve	1 serve	1 serve	1 serve
Digestive Biscuits With	2	2	2	2	2
Milk (3.25% fat)	1 cup	1 cup	1 cup	1 cup	1 cup
Lunch					
Soup	1 cup	1 cup	1 cup	1 cup	1 cup
Protein sandwich (1 serve = 2 slices white bread/ wholemeal bread) with 20g protein filling	2 serves	1 serve	1 serve	1 serve	1 serve
Afternoon Tea					
Plain Water Crackers with Cream Cheese: 1 serve = 2 crackers, 1 Tb cream cheese	1 serve	1 serve	1 serve	1 serve	1 serve
Plain Water Crackers with Cottage Cheese: 1 serve = 2 crackers, 1 Tb cottage cheese	1 serve	1 serve	1 serve	1 serve	1 serve
Plain Water Crackers with Cheese: 1 serve = 2 crackers, 20g cheese	1 serve	1 serve	1 serve	1 serve	1 serve
Digestive Biscuits	2	2	2	2	2
Dinner					
Protein Component	1 serve	1 serve	1 serve	1 serve	1 serve
Starch Component (potato, rice, kumara, mashed potato etc.)	½ cup	½ cup	½ cup	½ cup	½ cup
Allowed Low Roughage Vegetables	1/3 cup	1/3 cup	1/3 cup	1/3 cup	1/3 cup
Custard – Sugar Free Or Vanilla Pudding – Sugar Free Or Chocolate Pudding – Sugar Free	½ cup	½ cup	½ cup	½ cup	½ cup
Allowed Stewed Fruit, sugar free - drained	½ cup	½ cup	½ cup	½ cup	½ cup
Sugar Free Jelly Dessert	½ cup	½ cup	½ cup	½ cup	½ cup
Supper					
Plain Water Crackers with Cream Cheese: 1 serve = 2 crackers, 1 Tb cream cheese	1 serve	1 serve	1 serve	1 serve	1 serve
Plain Water Crackers with Cottage Cheese: 1 serve = 2 crackers, 1 Tb cottage cheese	1 serve	1 serve	1 serve	1 serve	1 serve
Plain Water Crackers with Cheese: 1 serve = 2 crackers, 20g cheese	1 serve	1 serve	1 serve	1 serve	1 serve
With Milk (Standard)	1 cup	2	2	2	2
Digestive Biscuits	2	1 cup	1 cup	1 cup	1 cup (250g)
* Once a day, 125g or ½ Cup of plain yoghurt					

Australian Male (with Diabetes)

Age Categories	40 – 49	50 – 59	60 – 69	70 – 79	80 +
Breakfast					
Porridge	1 cup	1 cup	1 cup	1 cup	1 cup
Cornflakes	1 cup	1 cup	1 cup	1 cup	1 cup
Ricies	1 cup	1 cup	1 cup	1 cup	1 cup
Stewed fruit (apple, pear, peaches) – sugar free, drained	½ cup	1/3 cup	1/3 cup	1/3 cup	1/3 cup
White Bread or Whole Meal Bread	2 slices	2 slices	1 slice	1 slice	1 slice
Margarine or Butter or Avocado Spread	2 tsp	2 tsp	1 tsp	1 tsp	1 tsp
Milk	½ cup	½ cup	½ cup	½ cup	½ cup
Low Calorie, Sugar Free Drink (Juice or Tea or Coffee etc.).	2/3 cup	2/3 cup	2/3 cup	2/3 cup	2/3 cup
Peanut Butter	2 Tb	2 Tb	2 Tb	2 Tb	2 Tb
Plain Yoghurt	½ cup	½ cup	½ cup	½ cup	½ cup
Morning Tea					
Plain Water Crackers with Cream Cheese: 1 serve = 2 crackers, 1 Tb cream cheese	1 serve	1 serve	1 serve	1 serve	1 serve
Plain Water Crackers with Cottage Cheese: 1 serve = 2 crackers, 1 Tb cottage cheese	1 serve	1 serve	1 serve	1 serve	1 serve
Plain Water Crackers, with Tuna: 1 serve = 2 crackers, 1 Tb Tuna	1 serve	1 serve	1 serve	1 serve	1 serve
Plain Water Crackers with Cheese: 1 serve = 2 crackers, 20g cheese	1 serve	1 serve	1 serve	1 serve	1 serve
Digestive Biscuits	4	4	2	2	2
With Milk (3.25% fat)	1 cup	1 cup	1 cup	1 cup	1 cup
Lunch					
Soup	1 cup	1 cup	1 cup	1 cup	1 cup
Protein sandwich (1 serve = 2 slices white bread/ wholemeal bread) with 20g protein filling	2 serves	2 serves	2 serves	2 serves	2 serves
Afternoon Tea					
Plain Water Crackers with Cream Cheese: 1 serve = 2 crackers, 1 Tb cream cheese	1 serve	1 serve	1 serve	1 serve	1 serve
Plain Water Crackers with Cottage Cheese: 1 serve = 2 crackers, 1 Tb cottage cheese	1 serve	1 serve	1 serve	1 serve	1 serve
Plain Water Crackers with Cheese: 1 serve = 2 crackers, 20g cheese	1 serve	1 serve	1 serve	1 serve	1 serve
Digestive Biscuits	4	4	4		2
Dinner					
Protein Component	1 serve	1 serve	1 serve	1 serve	1 serve
Starch Component (potato, rice, kumara, mashed potato etc.).	½ cup	½ cup	½ cup	½ cup	½ cup
Allowed Low Roughage Vegetables	1/3 cup	1/3 cup	1/3 cup	1/3 cup	1/3 cup
Custard – Sugar Free or Vanilla Pudding – Sugar Free or Sugar Free Chocolate Pudding	½ cup	½ cup	½ cup	½ cup	½ cup
Allowed Stewed Fruit, sugar free – drained	½ cup	½ cup	½ cup	½ cup	½ cup
Sugar Free Jelly	½ cup	½ cup	½ cup	½ cup	½ cup
Supper					
Plain Water Crackers with Cream Cheese: 1 serve = 2 crackers, 1 Tb cream cheese	1 serve	1 serve	1 serve	1 serve	1 serve
Plain Water Crackers with Cottage Cheese: 1 serve = 2 crackers, 1 Tb cottage cheese	1 serve	1 serve	1 serve	1 serve	1 serve
Plain Water Crackers with Cheese: 1 serve = 2 crackers, 20g cheese	1 serve	1 serve	1 serve	1 serve	1 serve
With Milk (3.25% fat)	1 cup	1 cup	1 cup	1 cup	1 cup
Digestive Biscuits	4	4	4	2	2
** once a day, 125g of plain yoghurt					

Feedback

"If you enjoyed this book, I'd be incredibly grateful if you could take a moment to leave a review. Your feedback helps other readers discover this story and supports my work as an author. Also, if you have suggestions on how to improve this book or possible topics to include in this book, please share your thoughts by clicking on the link below:

https://maximisednutrition.com/holistic-guide-feedback

This book is part of a series of books called, "Empower Series". The aim of this series is to empower you with both knowledge and practical information in holistic health so that you can live the best life you can.

Thank you,

Prem Nand, Clinical Dietitian – Nutritionist, NZRD.

Legal Disclaimer

This book provides helpful dietary advice for managing Diverticulitis and Diverticular Disease. It has been created by Maximised Nutrition Ltd (maximisednutrition.com).

By using this guide, you agree to the following terms. If you do not agree, please avoid using the content.

We have done our best to offer practical tips, but please remember, this information is not a substitute for personalized advice from a qualified healthcare professional. The author, a Registered Dietitian based in New Zealand, is also allowed to practice in Australia, but not in other countries, like the USA. So, if you are outside of these areas, consider this guide more of a general resource.
It is important to note that this book is not meant to replace medical care, and you should see a doctor if your symptoms do not improve. The information here is accurate as of the time it was written, but it might not cover every detail.

By using this book, you agree not to hold Prem Nand, Clinical Dietitian-Nutritionist, Maximised Nutrition Ltd, or any of its owners, agents, or employees responsible for any issues that come up from using this information, unless there has been gross negligence or intentional harm.

.If you have concerns about the content of this educational product, please send an e-mail (**publisher@maximisednutrition.com**) or write us at the following address:

Maximised Nutrition Limited
C/- Whangarei Wellness Centre, Level 1
25 Rathbone Street
Whangarei 0110, New Zealand

Made in the USA
Monee, IL
02 November 2026

67385349R00070